Your Body Really Can Heal Itself

Unleashing the Healing Miracle Within

Dr. Lucky's 7 Steps to Health & Longevity

Dr. Thomas Lucky

MEDICAL ADVICE DISCLAIMER

Printed in USA by Bexsi Publishing

Dedication

I would like to dedicate this book to my lovely wife Roxanne. From the very first day that we opened the clinic, she has been and continues to be a tremendous support every step of the way. Even though at times she may not feel acknowledged, she has been the operation center throughout the years. She is a wonderful wife and friend for whom I could not be grateful enough.

I also want to thank the following people who have helped me through the years: my mother and father, Rev. and Mrs. Wallace Lucky, for always believing in me, my Uncle "D" who helped make my education possible, and, of course, all the patients who were willing to tell their stories. I am also grateful to Rawson's Photography for my photographs of self and the CT scans, and Rev. Trent Allen for proofing the manuscript.

Dr. Thomas Lucky
tlucky_1@yahoo.com

Table of Contents

Foreword

By David Van Koevering
Co-inventor of the first musical synthesizer

⸺⸺◄◆►⸺⸺

As an international public speaker and a scientist with over 600-patented protected concepts, I met Dr. lucky several years ago in a conference where I was speaking.

His comments to me regarding ideas I had shared in my presentation regarding Quantum Healing and Quantum Physics rang true to me. I knew within a few minutes that his insight and experience with his patients were correct based on his great comprehensive understanding of the unseen or the invisible reality of quantum physics.

I have 40 years of history in this unseen world of electron subatomic particles and have spoken to scientists, medical professionals, and researchers worldwide.

My first encounter at that conference with Dr. Lucky was a most remarkable interaction. My wife Becky and I have since then shared many days with him discussing and developing protocols, procedures, and high tech instruments that he owned before meeting me, and now some of my inventions he has tested and is using them with successful results, including clinical tests that are positive.

I consider my friend, Dr. Lucky, and his assistant Majory McElroy, to be among a growing movement that is on the front edge of a revolution in the healing arts. The word revolution is rather overworked in science. The physicist Paul Davies has identified, nevertheless, that even those with a merely casual interest in scientific matters, will be aware that some truly revolutionary changes are taking place. We refer not so much to the specific discoveries that are happening all the time, nor just to the many wonderful advances in technology. True, these changes are revolutionary enough in themselves. There is, however, a far more profound transformation taking place in the underlying science itself in the way that scientists view their world.

Dr. Lucky has established his medical practice around this unique insight that is, in my observation, a specific paradigm! He views the role of healing of the human body not as a result of the doctors and medicines having the role to cause healing, rather that the body is created to heal itself, and the role of doctors and their correct use of drugs or supplements is only to help and assist the body to heal itself.

The philosopher Thomas Kuhn has argued that scientists build their conception of reality around certain specific paradigms. A paradigm is not a theory, but a framework of thought, a conceptual scheme around which the data of experiment and observation are organized. From time to time in the history of ideas, a shift occurs in the basic paradigm. When this happens, not only do the scientific theories change, but the scientist's conception of the world changes as well. This is what Dr. Lucky is demonstrating now. Consider the paradigm changes in this book. I know from the experience with thousands of my attendees, students, and readers worldwide, that you can hear more than I or Dr. Lucky can say. The Designers Code is in your body. Learn, know, comprehend, and accept the paradigm changes from these pages and be healed!

David Van Koevering

davidvankoevering.com

WARNING: This is an unconventional book and I would recommend the reader start with Chapter 8 and read about an unconventional topic in the medical field,

....Faith

Preface

The information in this book is the combination of all my training, conferences, and the hundreds of books I have read as well as my experience helping patients throughout my career. If you want to seek more information on some of the science that supports what I present herein, I recommend the following books:

- Quantum Mechanics: The Young Double Slit Experiment Copyright(c) 1998 by Gary Felder and Kerry Felder.
- Article from Live Science: Imaging of Ultraweak Spontaneous Photon Emission from Human Body Displaying Diurnal Rhythm Masaki Kobayashi, Daisuke Kikuchi, Hitoshi Okamura Plos One 4 (7); e6256.doi:10.1371/journal. pone. 0006356
- Energy Medicine The Scientific Basis James L. Oschman

There are certain doctors that have greatly influenced my life and I would like to thank them here:

Dietrich Klinghardt MD, Levels of healing in book

Jonathan Wright MD

Lee Cowden MD

Daniel Clark MD

Dr. Faye Gresham

My Wonderful Patients; they are the best doctors and teachers!

I want to say thank you to Lord Jesus Christ, my wife and family for their encouragement, the people who have come to me for help physically, Rev. Hugh and Margaret Davis, and Kathy H. (who helped me find the Clinic and keep it running), Majory and Bonnie (who have volunteered their precious time to support me at the clinic).

Team effort built our clinic that is not possible without all the players.

For those who want to know me better, I refer you to the following biblical passages:

1 Corinthians 1:27-28; for the best description about my clinic.

Roman 8:38; we are not tied to our past but should live in the present

Proverbs 23:7; for a man actually thinks from his heart.

Introduction

My whole life has been about rebellion and rejection of social norms. My disbelief in disease and diagnosis has caused much turmoil in my professional life. The word disease is really just that, dis-ease. The emotions and the body are not at ease, not at equilibrium and expressing that unhappiness through manifested illness. Once labeled as a certain medical disease it has a snowball effect on the emotions and heart of a patient who now tries to live down to it rather than live up to his full potential of health. If someone tells you that you have cancer, then you will start acting like a cancer patient soon to die instead of a person ready to get well. The curing of a disease tends to be more about making money off the patient, about insurance companies, and disempowering the patient.

I am about an entirely different approach to health and healing and the inevitable, longevity that results.

I believe in empowering people and removing labels that limit them from seeing themselves in a better, hopeful light. The body heals itself with removal of the label and proper nutritional supplementation. I have treated some of the sickest patients on the face of the Earth, people who come in their beds, with their last hope, last gasp of breath and ready to die. I do not use many of the things that traditional doctors use, and I do not treat the body alone. My methods are different from those used by traditional medical doctors. Healing is about treating the whole person, the heart, body, and soul, for only then can they fully heal. My goal is to educate the public that there are other methods available, methods which can dramatically improve one's health and lengthen their lives. I have written this book to tell the people outside of my reach that there are alternatives, there is hope and there are tangible healing results that I have witnessed throughout all of the years in my practice.

Let us start from the beginning of my story:

I grew up in Mississippi. Right off the bat I had some significant challenges in getting into elementary school, as I had a speech impediment. I would get sort of tongue tied, people could not understand me, and the only language I could manage was to stomp my feet, so I was delayed getting to school. Once at school, they did not like me particularly well. I constantly daydreamed in class, punctuated by my sudden jumping. The teachers begged my parents to put me into remedial classes, and informed them that I needed a CT of my brain to find the origin of my behavior. What they did not realize was that while I was daydreaming, the other kids would prick me with a pin. Being really shy, I was afraid to talk or do anything about it, so in the second grade they put me into a slow learning class for the mentally retarded.

Children in my class picked on me all the way to 5th grade, but that is when the tables turned. I had developed a real anger problem, and on seeing how tall I was getting, and my newfound long arms, I decided to fight back and began beating up every boy in the class. I went from feeling constantly victimized to beating up one person that became one of the best wrestlers in the state of Mississippi. During one fight, I even stuck his head in the toilet. Being a bully gave me a feeling of power, but also brought me to the point where I was so angry that I decided to try to fail the 5th grade by making straight zeros for half a year.

Fortunately, my parents saw that I was just manipulating things, and halfway through the year I changed my mind when I received my salvation. My father had predicted that this would happen. I went from being a horrible student to a very good one, pulling all my classes up to straight A's (except English, which gave me difficulty all the way through college). I still maintained my rebellious streak, though, and that is actually, what got me to what I am doing today.

I had already set up a pattern, however, one that kept wrecking my life. I would view myself as stupid, take the hardest classes available in high school and college just to prove myself stupid, then make it through with the highest scores in the class, often by finding shortcuts through the problems and avoiding the messy complicated ways that teachers and the system demanded I solve them.

I went into advanced biology and took the highest level of Science you could possibly take at our school. The principal and teacher looked at me and said, *"You don't need to be in this class, you need to take JROTC. You will fail this class, and you can get your credits and graduate by taking JROTC. You have no chance in passing this class."* I replied, *"This is Advanced Biology; this is what I like to do."* I ended up making the highest grade in the class, so when the principal had to give me the award, he said, *"You know something? We were confused. It was not you. It was another Lucky that we were thinking about."* That pattern went through medical school all the way to residency.

I always believed that it was the result that mattered, not the formality of how you got there. I was a frustration to all my teachers, and probably myself as well, even though in the end I would graduate with honors.

The fact that I have a sort of photographic memory made things even worse in college. I would read the books, skip the classes, and just take the tests, passing with flying colors. If the teacher forced me to attend class, I would just fall asleep because I had already read everything and knew what the teacher was going to say. I started out in chemical engineering, but did not like the lab work or the time the classes met. I did my usual by going home, memorizing the books, and rarely going to class. Not the brightest thing to do... not attending the classes in your major. I was also taking classes in biology, zoology, histology, molecular genetics, and others that had nothing to do with chemical engineering.

Things changed when I had to take my grandpa and great uncle to the doctor. I became concerned with their health issues and that interested me in medicine. I still did not attend class very often and once was so bored I fell asleep during a test. Dr. Morrow scored me in the 60s on that test, until I went back and showed him everything in the book, explained my answers and shortcuts. I came away from that with a perfect score. I guess I was just too rebellious and bored to learn things in the way they wanted me to. The result was that I avoided the typical educational brain washing. In the end, I graduated from Mississippi State University with honors before entering the University of Mississippi Medical Center.

My big danger at this point was falling asleep in class. Still, I managed to make it through and into the clinical years.

Throughout medical school and residency, I was rebellious, always questioning authority. Any time a case came in where the attending physician gave a simple solution for a patient's condition, I would question it. I'd see some detail that matched up to some obscure condition I'd read in one of my text books, would be right, and end up saving someone's life as a result.

In one case it was the attending physician saying it was cancer, while I'd spotted the fact that the patient slept with his dogs and so it must be Rocky Mountain Spotted Fever in the bone marrow; the first such case ever. A CDC associate stated, "I should publish the case." We did CT scans, colonoscopy, upper endoscopy, bone marrow, flow cytometry, all kinds of work for folic acid deficiency. He presented a temperature of 104 degrees, mental status changes, severe pancytopenia, hyponatremia, and liver function abnormalities. He was bleeding out his mouth, but they did not look at the obvious which was the tick. He was sleeping with dogs and he had ticks on himself. He did not have a rash but not every case presents as a rash. I immediately started the patient on doxycycline against the other doctors' wishes and his issues resolved quickly. If you do not treat it, **Rickettsial** illness is a medical emergency.

We spend time and listen to our client, not running them through like cattle. My motto is to look always at the patient not just the lab or you could end up with a dead patient.

I am a mixture of everybody that I have ever gone and listened to, and do not do anything that anyone in particular does. I listen to what people say and come up with my own way of solving the problem, just as I always have since childhood. As a result, hospital staff screamed, ridiculed me, and I made ER doctors cry.

I question conventional medical wisdom constantly, because in my opinion the patient's health is the most important part about medicine, not the physician's ego.

One doctor would diagnose a patient with a stroke, only to have me recognize the problem as being a magnesium deficiency. Once the patient began to recover under my treatment, I verbally landed into the other doctor. I did not have patience for such things. I have angered hospitals and medical facilities from coast to coast, and was not always the easiest person to get along with in the past.

I used to look at things this way. I was egotistical and everything revolved around me. Before I graduated from Residency, the Assistant Dean called me into his office and said that I had the most complaints from staff and doctors, but then told me something that changed my life! He said, *"Life is not always about being right even though you are right."* He told me because of the long hours and dedication I had for patient care I was a doctor's doctor but I would burn out if I continued at my pace. I received a bottle of my favorite supplement from him at graduation: Magnesium.

I am much more amicable now, although I am still learning, still teaching myself, and still rebelling against conventional wisdom and medical diagnoses brought about by plain laziness. I have learned that I am really only a witness of the miracle within anyone who is willing to unleash it. Each of us is the blueprint for healing but God does the healing.

I am a minister now, and have my own clinic and enjoy seeing clients all over the United States and the World, spending several hours with every single one because my desire is to see them well, and I love seeing the miracles that often result. Medicine for me is fun, not just a job but also an integral part of my life. To see people go from desperate and hopeless, to walking, running, playing, and living again, is what completes my life. To find out more about my clinic, go to www.christcenteredcare.com.

Flowood Lifestyle and Wellness Clinic employs on three levels of healing: the Physical, the Emotional, and the Spiritual. The three integrate, one affecting the other, so we treat the whole holistically. If you only heal the body and there is a concern that still occupies your heart, or a past event that yet lies heavily upon your spirit, then you will not heal, you will stay sick for the rest of your life. Only when you get to the larger issues that have been causing the physical problems will true and complete healing take place.

When I first meet the patient, instead of asking them questions about their health problems I tell them what is wrong. I tell them all of the significant events that ever happened in their life including when they were in the womb as well as significant events that happened in their ancestors' lives, their parents, and grandparents. They are amazed and confirm everything that I told them as true. I then elaborate and give them all the details and missing pieces of the puzzlWe are all made of energy, both our physical bodies and emotions. We emanate energy, make it flash on and off and, like an electrician, fixes a broken circuit. I, too, repair the energy circuit of a patient. In essence, I called myself an electrician for a human being. When your circuits are broken we repair them, and once your circuits are right then you get well and do not even know what happens.

I had a lady recently who was in kidney failure and very swollen with edema. When she got in my office, she said, *"I don't know what's going on in this place. You haven't done anything but I've been to the bathroom six times."* I said that I did not know what was going on either, but the next day she was well. She did not have any swelling whatsoever. Now she is telling everybody about me and I did not physically do anything to her.

What I do is akin to brainwashing a patient with hope, and healing the hopeless feeling within their heart. It is their own bodies that start the healing. What the heart believes, the body can do!

I have various equipments in my practice but I have gotten to the point of just using my hands to detect the energy flow and blockages. I can tell if a person has any abnormal cells in his body. I see the signs. Your body will tell you everything that has ever happened in your life, if you know how to listen. **It is nothing psychic, just educated observation.**

My methods are about compassion, empathy, and patience. Healing is not about diagnosing, labeling, and taking expensive medications. It is about humor, it is about listening to yourself, discovering what is inside, and freeing yourself from the troubles keeping you sick. I work together with my patients, even if I have to call them daily or make 500-mile house calls to see them. We are a team, and I will do whatever it takes to help my teammate recover from what ails him, whether it's physical or not.

I am not against my fellow doctors, and not fighting the system. I simply want everyone to know that there is more to medicine than is commonly practiced. With the right attitude, you can perform what seem to be miracles. Thus, vantage point is crucial. Instead of having cancer, you simply have abnormal cells. You are not old, for we associate old people with illness and short life ahead. You are instead young, always young: 30 years young, 50 years young, and 70 years young! You do not have a disease, for a disease implies a contract that you must take, a lacking of something the body requires or a belief in your heart with which your body is negatively interacting. You have a very treatable condition.

It is very important to remember always that beliefs can kill or cure. Body, Emotion, and Spirit are one. Believe you can get better and you will! Believe you are young and you will remain so! Dwelling on past fears can sicken you. Looking forward to future ailments can also sicken you. Always bring yourself to stay in the Present as the famous but wise saying calls for in Latin: Carpe Diem (Seize the Moment). Recognize problems, but perceive them as obstacles to overcome, to solve and to resolve rather than crises to dwell on. The key is to deal with the obstacles and move on with your life.

" *There is only one cause of unhappiness: the false beliefs you have in your head, beliefs so widespread, so commonly held, that it never occurs to you to question them.* "

-Anthony De Mello

Chapter ONE

7 Beliefs That Are Killing You

A belief is a shared truth. It is some idea that a person or a collective of people determine as being true. However, a belief can also be a lie. A falsehood that people nonetheless cling to continually. These are lies that often can lead people astray. We simply pass down most beliefs without questioning its origin or continued relevance. Many beliefs rob us of control over our lives and our health. In either case, belief can have powerful consequences, and is in fact a major component of what I address with my patients.

A belief can heal or harm. Believe that your life is coming to an end in eight days and you will not even try to prevent it. Your subconscious will do everything it can to make it come true. On the other hand, believe that you can get over some illness that has been plaguing you, and even conventional medical practice agrees that is at least half the battle. Belief has started wars, won causes, and both created and cured large-scale suffering.

Belief is a powerful thing, particularly for your health. What you think, what you believe, your body will react to. If you believe yourself sick, then you will end up sick as a result. We all need to believe in something, so why not believe in something positive?

You are probably asking, "Why would anyone want to believe themselves sick? Who would ever do that?" You would be surprised, because beliefs and their consequences can be tricky and slip under your conscious radar. I have compiled a list of seven beliefs that you may not realize could be killing you right now. Let us look at them.

1. I have to suffer to be closer to God

I am a Christian, a minister in fact, so I know much about this one, and many of my patients are faithful Christians as well. Many of them know where in the Bible it says that Paul had to have a thorn in his side and asked to get it removed 3 times, but God did not do it. With this biblical precedent, they conclude that sometimes we must first suffer for God in order to be well. My personal belief, though, is that we do not have to suffer for God. He is bigger than that! He loves us!

The Holy Bible says in III John 1:2 KJV, *"Beloved I wish **above all things** that thou mayest prosper and be in health, even as your soul prospereth."* In other words, you prosper in being healthy even as your soul prospers. This is in direct opposition to the belief that you have to live in suffering that God may favor you. He gets more glory when people are well and are able to be better people that they may show their light to this world.

Think about it from the point of view of a parent. As a parent, would you want your children to go out of their way to suffer for you? Of course not! Well, we are God's children, so how do you think he feels every time someone tortures himself in His name?

What is happening here is that people are recreating the sacrifice that Jesus made on the cross. However, Jesus made his sacrifice so that we would not need to do so ourselves. He died so that we may live and be free of our own self-imposed suffering. The suffering that we insist on committing upon ourselves in the name of this false belief is what hinders us from our healing process.

In order to heal or better ourselves, we need to believe that we can. How, then, are we to do if our belief steers us in the exact opposite direction? It is contradictory.

People believe that they have to mimic this grand sacrifice made by the Son of God in order to seek His approval, but I ask you, are you the Son of God? No! Then why are you trying to replicate a sacrifice He made so that we would not have to? This belief leads people to punish themselves every time they start to feel themselves too healthy or too successful. Some have even taken this to the extreme by eating junk on the premise that, *"Well, I have to suffer and die anyway, it might as well be on junk food"*.

Humankind is not preordained to suffer. Genetics comprise only about ten percent of the illnesses; the other 90 percent is your own responsibility. Inheritance of such conditions is an excuse for not being able to do anything about the situation. We like to play the victim or blame our circumstance. If you resign yourself to self-sacrifice, you give this responsibility to someone else. People who will take advantage of your desire to suffer through selling you expensive products you do not really need.

So, what are you to do? Let us start by defining God.

Maybe you think that God is out to punish people because he is a father figure to you, and as a child, your own father was abusive. Many people subconsciously equate God to pain and punishment, because that is what they suffered at the hands of parents, teachers, and other authority figures during their formative years. You need to understand what God really is to you, and see if there is an error in your beliefs about him.

Once you recognize where your viewpoint really comes from, then you can insert a new one: a viewpoint in which God loves you and wants you to get well, to better your life. Once you see this, you can get well.

2. I am not worthy to be healthy

Many people believe they are not worthy of being healthy, as if it is some divine right that no human should have. However, the Bible says that God made man in his image, so how could we not be worthy of being heal. You established your personality by the age of seven; that is who you are for the rest of your life. If your father did not treat you right, told you that you would never be good, never succeed, then that is your established self-viewpoint by the age of seven. You believe your program cannot change regardless how much you try. You cannot possibly succeed, so you put yourself in situations where you cannot. If you have been programmed with the belief that you are not worth anything, can never make anything, and are already a failure, you will have a very hard time believing in yourself and leading a balanced life on the notion that you are not good enough. You are not good enough as a life partner, not good enough to be successful, not good enough to be happy and healthy.

This program will loop through your heart the rest of your life, although it did not even originate with you. Someone else who played a crucial role in your childhood, usually your parent(s) imbedded it into your sub-consciousness. Your grandparents programmed your parents with burdens passed down to you and the scheme goes on to generations back to childhoods of their ancestors and will carry forward to your children unless the cycle is broken.

Our false belief that we are not worthy of success or health stems directly from someone else, not from the Divine.

The solution? Value yourself.

You feel unworthy because you do not love yourself, and you feel that way because as a child you did not feel enough love directed at you. All fathers love their children, but very few of them actually say, *"I love you"* to their children. A simple phrase that maybe the father feels would compromise his manliness if it escaped his lips, but a very important phrase for the developing child. Yet, this simple phrase is a powerful thing, and its lack can set you up into a belief system where you feel unworthy your entire life.

Remember, the issues in your life affect the issues in your tissues. Feel unworthy and your body will comply. Most people go to a doctor to feel their worth, to hear the diagnosis then the treatment, which ends up being the penance they must do in order to feel worthy of being healthy, to feel they have value. This method, of course, comes at a large monetary cost, which goes back to people's need to suffer.

A far easier and more valuable solution is to tell yourself how much worth you have. Stand before a mirror, look yourself straight in the eye, then tell yourself *"I love you"*. Say this aloud and do not move from looking straight at yourself. It will be surprisingly hard, but it is the start that you need. Address every part of your body and thank it for being there and doing its job. Then tell yourself why you have value, and write yourself a letter listing your accomplishments. State how you have affected other people for the better, and the plans you have to better yourself and improve the lives of others in your small corner of the Universe. Then go out and see how you can continue to improve your situation and love yourself all the more.

You must see that you have worth as an individual in order to be healthy.

3. I don't deserve to be healthy

Once you feel worth as a person, the next closely related step is to feel that you deserve to be healthy. You might feel enough self-worth, but despite that, you could still feel that you do not deserve good health. You have not done enough good deeds yet. Or... why should you be healthy when your friends are not? If your friends or other people are not healthy then what sets you apart that you deserve it so much better?

Now imagine the other guy you are talking about. He is saying the exact thing about himself that *he* does not deserve to get healthy because *you* are not healthy. This is a self-defeating premise that can spread like a plague. Just as before, if you believe you do not deserve to be healthy, then your body will comply.

Most doctors heal the separate parts of the body, but I deal with the person holistically. There was an Army Study in which they removed white blood cells from someone and sent them to California in a petri dish while the subject remained on the other side of the country. Researcher had the subject to watch a movie or something stimulating, and recorded the activity in the white blood cells at the same time. The result was that the cells had a simultaneous reaction as the subject, even though thousands of miles separated them! White blood cells contain receptors on their membranes for emotional neurotransmitters such as dopamine and cortisol and they have endocannabinoids (CB2) receptors that also regulate emotions. There is a whole science behind this phenomenon called Psychoneuroimmunoendocrinology that describes the connection between the psyche (brain), the peripheral nervous system, the immune system, and the endocrine system.

The case of one of my patients, Lee B., also demonstrates non-local simultaneous healing. When she stopped blaming herself for her son not talking, the back problem immediately resolved and her son's problems with speaking resolved. He began talking at that same moment of her healing, even though he was over 200 miles away.

The environment around you and yourself connects to "all that is", God. Believe you can heal, that you deserve healing, and you will. However, believe you do not deserve healing and the body will not. The body can heal anything if you believe that it can and give it the support it needs. Feed it fear and anxiety, and your health will only worsen.

Healing comes from inside our bodies, not externally. Only when you recognize that you are ready to be healed will the healing begin. Then nothing will stop that process.

4. I have to exchange something to achieve health

Exchange is the basis for everything in this world. That goes for sacrifice as well. People need to exchange something just like God did with His Son. You exchange money, you exchange time, and you always exchange something to get something else. This belief in exchange goes back to the duality of Creation that since Good exists therefore so does Evil. If something good must happen, then so must something bad, therefore in order to attain good health you will go out of your way to expect something unpleasant to happen.

Once again, if you expect something bad to happen, if you believe that it must, then it surely will.

God only created Good, not Evil. He created abundance, light, and health. He did not make poverty, darkness, or sickness, so why would he demand something of you in exchange for your God-given right to better health? People negatively focus on the worst-case scenario waiting for the second boot to drop.

Think of the people you meet on a daily basis. How many of them will tell you about some great thing that happened to them that day, be it big or small? Now how many of them will launch into complaints about the smallest disruption to their lives and go out of their way to spread the negativity around? It is this focus on the negative that keeps people suspicious about anything really good, about a "free lunch". They will focus on the one missing piece in an otherwise complete 5000 piece puzzle, instead of looking at the beauty of the rest of the whole.

Focus on the positive, and you will attract the positive. Too many times people feel a need to exchange something for their improved health or think they do not deserve of it in the first place that only attracts more consequences that are negative.

This might be more difficult than it seems. We are so accustomed to focusing on the negative that thinking positive is actually something that gets one ridiculed. However, there are ways to start.

One of the most effective things I do is to perform contract shredding. People do not understand when they go to the doctors and get a diagnosis that they have to sign a contract. Usually a contract requires an exchange of something. It is power! There are penalties to breaking contracts, and when you go to the doctor, you pay money to see that doctor. Let us suppose that doctor gives you a diagnosis of Diabetes. You just received everything that doctor has to offer for Diabetes, which is heart attack, stroke, amputations, blindness, kidney failure, dialysis, and the list goes on. The doctor then says, *"We can't really do anything about this other than slow the progression."* By the way, I know this is **not** true and you **can** reverse the progress of anything!

You can make a contract about anyone or anything including weight release. We have to be careful what we sign. I have to warn people all the time when they fill out their intake forms, to make sure they know what they are signing.

When clients sign our contract we offer them hope, choice, and the empowerment of themselves. When one makes a contract, the body is actually going back and researching the memory of what happened that allows the healing to take place, so if you break these contracts and you shred these contracts you can immediately free people of all kinds of issues. They free themselves because they are no longer in debt to the errant contract.

I am not against doctors. This is not a fight against the system, as far as I am concerned. Doctors are kind. They work hard. They work to see 60 patients per day. But they have what I call psychological glaucoma that means they see through tunnel vision so they cannot see what is going on in the periphery and they do not accept it until it actually gets into their visual field. Yet, there are miracles happening all around them. They say the miracles are simply spontaneous remission. If that is the case, we frequently see spontaneous remission at our clinic.

A young lady in her 60's had gas discomfort and thought she had a viral or bacterial infection. She had already scheduled an appointment with a GI doctor to see what was going on. She was also fatigued and had some vague chest discomfort. We did some colon work and discussed a land issue and her family situation. The symptoms resolved without further problems. She decided to get an ultrasound, from which the doctor stated she had gallstones and ordered a HIDA scan and placed her on PPI. At this time, she was having no symptoms and I did not believe she needed the test. She decided to do the test and the report indicated she had mildly reduced ejection fraction on the Gall Bladder and the number the doctor told her was severe. I called the Radiologist and he stated she had severe acalculus cholecystitis and needed immediate surgical consult. I explained that someone was not telling the truth! One doctor said she had gallstones and another one states acalculus that means no gallstones. The radiology report indicated severe decrease function of the gallbladder but the description indicated it was only mild and possibly biliary dyskinesia.

The moral to this story is; always get every lab, x-ray, and pathology report and keep a record of it because it could save your life. The result was that the lady only needed hydrochloric acid for hypochlorohydia. She did not need surgery. Her contracts with the physicians needed to be shredded. She is now totally asymptomatic and if she develops gallstones in the future, we will work on removing them without surgery.If an overweight man wants to trim some fat, that's a good thing. But tell him he has to *lose* weight and the semantics get him every time. Losing something is always unpleasant and to be avoided. You can lose a husband, lose your kids, lose money. Instead, he needs to *release* his excess weight, let it go in a healthy way. This is only a minor change in semantics, but one which gets away from the expectation of "exchange" and away from the fear and anxiety that accompanies it.

Society programs people with such expectations as only living to about 70 years of age, based either on current scientific wisdom or on some quote from the Bible that may be either taken out of context or not applicable anymore. They expect no more than 70 years and so they convince their bodies to start shutting down around age 65. Yet, there are people living past 100 years young right now with no reason not to live longer. You just have to drop your errant expectations…the need to have a good life in exchange for a short one.

Many of my techniques employ on quieting the heart and removing one's fears. You do not need to exchange anything to be well; you just need to quiet the disruptive thoughts in your heart and be well naturally because your body wants to be. Quiet the heart and replace the negative thoughts with life enhancing positive ones, and allow the body to transform itself. No major exchange needed, and no need to feel guilty about "getting something for nothing".

After all, aren't the best things in life free?

5. I am not lovable as I am.

"I am" is a very powerful phrase. It has to do with being in the present, the here and now. In general, people do not feel loved due to some circumstance that happened in their lives and that makes them unhappy. This is because the past is the "I was", and this changes moment to moment. They feel unlovable right now because of something in the past, yet that feeling allows their past to destroy their present and future.

The Bible says, *"Now is the accepted time; behold, now is the day of salvation,"* not the past or the future. The Bible also says that God is All Powerful, All Knowing, and Always Present. He is in the "Now" and acts upon us in the "Now". Thus the key is to be in the Now. In order to be healed or to have your body changed; you must be in the Now. You cannot change the Past, and the Future is simply waiting to become the Present in a short time, so you must pay attention to the Present. It matters not how lovable or unlovable you may have been "back then", you are in the "now".

How lovable are you right now?

That is entirely up to you. Your answer to that question is not based upon your anxiety over the Past, not on how stressed you are (for the stress follows the mood not the other way around), but on your ability to recognize that you are a loved person. Do this, and realize as well that you can be in the moment of "I am", which is always changing, and you do not have to fear. You can quiet yourself, and radiate the love in your life. Then you can let your body do its work.

You ask, *"What if I have no friends? Then how can I be lovable?"* Remember that God is here in the Present; you are his child, a part of His body, Therefore, God loves you. There is an abundance of love but you need to know where to look. God made you in his likeness, and he has placed you on this plane of human experience to realize this abundant Love. God is of Love, you are a part of God and therefore you are of Love. God loves you because you are a part of him. Your arm is a part of you and you take care of it, but let us say a fire burns your arm. Then you would nurture it even more because you want it to get better. Your arm learns through that painful experience not to come near fire. Likewise, we learn through our life experiences. We get hurt both physically and emotionally, not because God wants us to suffer but because he wants us to learn and grow through our experiences and become more intimately acquainted with his abundant Love.

It is a problem that can twist back upon itself. You want to change your body, improve yourself so that you can become lovable, but you will not improve until you see yourself as lovable. A conundrum that can be hard to escape, so how should you go about it?

The answer is quite simple.

Being lovable is a choice, *your* choice.

We often ask Google or Bing to search for something. Similarly, our bodies are always searching for information that we have input into our minds. The Bible states in Matthew 21:22 *"And all things, whatsoever ye shall ask in prayer, believing, ye shall receive."* We focus on why are we so fat, why are we so poor, why are we so sick, etc. As a result, that is what our Google (computer search engine of the body) returns. We focus on the negative instead of the positive…what we lack instead of what we have in abundance.

So…are you lovable?

6. It is not okay to do what it takes to be well.

This goes back to self worth and not loving yourself enough to have your priorities aright. People spend their lives working hard to make money, sacrifice everything for their family, exchange everything in their lives for money, then in the last two weeks of their lives spend it all and everyone else's fortune on their health because they did not pay enough attention to it as they went along. They end up not wanting to do what it takes to get well because they are thinking, *"Well, I'm going to die soon anyway."* Yet the real reason they "die soon" is because they expected it and therefore refused to do what they needed to keep their health.

Actually, the brain does not hear the word 'not', therefore when you say, *"I will, I'll try, I can,"* the body automatically puts in the word 'not' because in childhood all we heard was "no, no, no," and that is why we do not try to do anything. To choose means to be empowered and God is always giving a person choice and from the beginning of the foundation of this earth, he gave us choice. Choice is free will and free agency.

You need to learn to do things differently, to get out of your rut. Do not waste any more precious time. Do not spend your entire life letting your health get worse and worse until it is too late. You really can take care of your health and still tend to the needs of your family. You just need to exercise *both* halves of your brain to find a way. Interject some creativity into your life and you will think up creative solutions that will allow you to have your cake and eat it too (Otherwise, what is the use in baking it in the first place?).

No one can ever force you into a given situation; you *always* have a choice. You do not need to choose between Money and Health, but rather find a way to keep both. The bible reveals that even Satan was given the freedom to choose, so why should *you* not be able to choose?

Feeling that it is not okay to do whatever it takes to be well stems from others saying that it is simply not acceptable. We want to stay healthy, but we do not want to take the responsibility to do what it takes. Science teaches us that the body is in a steady state of decline after the age of 25, so in the back of our hearts we sincerely believe this, and decide not even to try. This assumption comes back to bite you in the rear when later you find yourself in a hospital hooked up to a respirator.

Okay so how do I change?

Question your belief systems. All of them! And if it is a belief you already questioned and fixed about 10 years back, then it is time to question it again. Beliefs may have changed for you since then. Question any assumed expectations that limit you, and then do whatever it takes to get well.

7. The body needs help to heal itself

If this is true, then how did humankind ever get well before medicine came around?

The body is always either trying to heal itself or to keep itself healthy. Cuts in skin heal by themselves, the liver has the ability to regenerate, and hair regrows. However, when we put boundaries on ourselves (boundaries imposed by a collective belief into which we trap ourselves), then we end up becoming our own self-fulfilling prophecy and we do not heal.

If you go to some doctors, the first thing established is that the doctor has all the power and you are unimportant. You sit down in the chair looking up at him. This position places you in an inferior position to which the subconscious lovingly clings. You are then open to whatever recommendations the doctor gives you. You believe the doctor when he tells you that you need certain medications or that what you have is incurable. However, that does not mean that it is incurable or lifelong bondage to medications. In fact, the body itself is the best curative.

I have seen many "incurable" patients that have gone from deathbed to healthy and walking. It is because their belief system was far more positive than others' in their situations were. Skin regenerates, heals on its own, so why then do we believe that the body cannot heal deeper scars as well? It is because our inability to believe this is possible is cluttering up the computer of our heart, holding back the process.

Messages and advertisements about medical products or services constantly barrage us that we "need", that we must have in order to be healthy. Belief in oneself gives a distant back seat to more commercial needs. If you go to a doctor for your high blood pressure and the doctor tells you that you will have to be on a medication for the rest of your life, then the doctor did not really do a thing. He just created an atmosphere of fear and submission based on the diplomas hanging on his wall and a wealth of superior-sounding attitude.

As I stated previously, I am not against the medical field. There is a place for medicine, but I think the medical field needs revamping to include alternative methods. Going to someone that believes in the body's own healing is a good first step. I know many people who come into my clinic hypertensive and plagued with all kinds of issues that now have no further need for medications, or even supplements. The point here is that the majority of everything is curable, but the only thing that can do this is the human body and its ability to cure itself.

Now if you broke your neck or something like that, then that is where a good doctor can come in, but they must also recognize that they are merely assisting the body, that *it* is the primary physician.

I speak from experience because I suffered a broken back and neck.

My wife and I were on our way home after taking our little dog from the Vet, when our Toyota sped out of control. Before we knew it, we had flipped three times with the top of the car coming down on my head each time. The accident knocked me unconscious, left my hair on the top of car, bleeding and living in the seventh heaven. Our car threw my wife and dog out the window and she hit her head on a tree flying by. She woke me from my stupor and told me that we just had a car wreck. I went from enjoying a dreamy fishing trip to being in severe back pain…the worse pain I have ever had in my life.

X-ray depicted that I had three fractures in my neck and three fractures in my back. God blessed me that my fractures were non-displaced but the health care establishment stated it usually takes 16 weeks to heal a fracture. We performed many procedures that we do at our clinic, and within five days after the accident, they could not find anything on multiple X-ray views. In fact, the doctor said there is no way a fracture could have been there in the first place. I refused pain meds after the first bout that made me see ants coming out of the ceiling, and two weeks later drove 1500 miles to Florida and back with a C-collar, without pain or pain medicine.

What was my treatment regimen?

I performed micro current therapy on myself, used the Ondamed machine the day I got out of the hospital, and had about twenty degrees of rotation of my neck. Five minutes after using the Ondamed, I was able to circumrotate my neck seventy degrees without difficulty. I used heavy glyconutrients, essential oils, reflexology, relaxation therapy, infrared light therapy, phototherapy, the Zyto machine, and of course Present Therapy for emotional issues. I woke up every night around 11:00 pm repeatedly experiencing the car wreck, and just prior to going to Florida for the medical conference I revisited the site of wreck, and have had no further flashbacks. Heart rate variability studies noted no decreased progress regarding increased sympathetic stress. About three years later, I had a thermogram performed by a doctor, and he looked at my records and then at my thermogram and said you are a self-healer. I told him I could not heal anything and only God was the healer. He could not believe I had no thermography pattern suggesting injury.

The doctor had one belief…that fractures take a long time to heal. I had an alternate belief. I refused to let his belief overrun my own.

Doctors are good in *assisting* the body to cure itself. As long as it is someone to help you clear the clutter and keep focused, and someone who will not overrun your own beliefs. If a doctor says, your condition is incurable and the best you can hope for is slowing it down. You must strengthen your belief system or find someone who is open to possibilities. The body has its own desire to be healthy, no matter what a given doctor might believe.

Beliefs can hold you back or beliefs can propel you to the highest heights. Beliefs can prevent our bodies from flushing the toxins that are damaging it. Beliefs can put unnecessary obstacles between you and perfect health.

Did you know that your body has an internal inherent memory system that you cannot control consciously? The body wants to survive and it will allow things to happen to it to prolong actually the time so you can come up with a solution to fix it. When we have a disease label, it indicates nothing more than that there is a condition of the body that continued and got into a desperate situation.

So what should you do about these false beliefs?

You must start by removing all the obstacles (these issues and beliefs) because many times the beliefs hold within them toxic chemicals that are keeping you sick. The body is sitting there desiring to live, reproduce and be plentiful, but it needs your help.

There are two basic purposes of a human and human body in this life. One is to live spiritually, physically, and mentally, and the other one is reproduction. If you do not live, you cannot reproduce, and if you do not reproduce, you do not live.

When excess programs bog your computer down and cause it to run slowly, you take it through a process of defragmentation that organizes and frees up space on the hard drive. Likewise, if you clean up the beliefs that are not serving you well, and then your body can heal. Here is a suggestion to help you defrag your beliefs. Get rid of your television. The only thing that is good on TV is maybe some old movie or the Weather Channel, and sometimes I wonder about the Weather Channel.

Because their stories are so profound, some of my patients have allowed me to include them in this book. We will be going through their cases throughout the book. First, you will see the description of a problem, followed by my comments on their case from the medical point of view.

The Case Of Lee B.

―――――――――◼◆◻――――――――

Dr. Lucky helped me in so many different ways. When I went to see him, I was taking medications from a regular doctor, my hair was falling out, I was tired, under active, weak, and hurting in the chest and heart. A friend from church recommended him and so I went to see him.

He ordered some blood-work consisting of a metabolic panel, did a test, then asked me some questions. We talked about me, and about my son, who was going to a speech therapist because he could not talk well at 2 years of age.

Dr. Lucky gave me a bottle of laser-treated water to drink and put me on a special diet to detoxify me. He also switched me off the regular meds to a natural herbal medication called Armor, as well as several supplements, calcium, vinegar, and some multivitamins.

I had been blaming myself for my son's speech problems, and Dr. Lucky helped me face this issue. I forgave myself for that and later, not only did my heart begin to heal, but also when I went home later that day, my son began talking like he never had!

He also told me that I had issues with a family member (which I had not even told him about!) He helped me face this issue, forgive that person, and soon afterwards my bloody bowels were healed.

Before I left from my first appointment, I told Dr. Lucky about some X-rays a chiropractor did that had found scoliosis. The chiropractor had treated me with little results, so Dr. Lucky took a look. He ran a finger down my back and something moved. Another X-Ray showed that it had all cleared up. I was so much better when I drove home.

Dr. Lucky is a very caring, understanding person who listened to my entire story. He mentions God frequently, and prayer is a regular part of his treatment. He checks up on me often, calling me when he is concerned about my family life. Thanks to the treatment I received, I am now doing much better.

The Doctor's Notes:

This case illustrates non-local healing at the same time the patient received her own healing. Lee stated that we helped her in so many different ways (marriage, health etc.) The amazing thing here is that when she first came to our office, her 2 year old son could only say "mama" clearly and a few other unintelligible words. She was taking him to speech therapy but did not see any improvement. She blamed herself for him not talking, and I told her *"First, let's get rid of that belief which is not yours anyway."* She cleared the belief and nothing seemed to really change, but as we were ending the visit she also told me she had been seeing a chiropractor who did an X-ray and had found scoliosis. He had treated her but did not see much results. I just ran my finger down her back to the L4-5 area and she told me she felt her back move. I told my wonderful helper, Bonnie, to assist me photographing her back and showed it to her and she stated it had not previously been like that.

So what happened? How was the back aligned? When she got over blaming herself for her son's delayed speech development, her back not only resolved, but her son also began talking, even though he was at home over 200 miles away at the time of her visit in my office. We see here that beliefs that are not serving us can hinder other people in our lives. Once we release the false belief, then miracles can take place in others and us that had been in bondage to our false beliefs.

❝ *As a man thinks in his heart, so is he* **❞**

-Proverbs 23:7 KJV Holy Bible

Chapter TWO

7 Strategies Towards Responsible Thinking

⋯⋯◄▶⋯⋯

If you want to be a responsible thinker, if you want to think clearly all the time, then there are some things you need to do to keep the body and brain in shape. I have summarized what you need to do in seven steps. Simple things you can do that will cost you no money yet greatly benefit you in life.

1. Committing to and Setting Boundaries

People who come to my clinic have various reasons for not getting well, and sometimes they even have ulterior motives. They come to me because their wife or female counterpart wanted them to and they are really expecting to fail, or they are here because someone had paid them to come. Maybe they like to have a disease title that is all their own, their way of having identity. They take possession by saying things like "my diabetes". An entity that has become all their own and now they are afraid of what would happen if they lost the label. Could they also handle losing the attention that the disease title brings?

I tell people, *"You must purge your heart of the negative programs to be well."* When I knew a person that has difficulty making decisions, he usually has low self-esteem issues and a desire to please everyone, but in the process does not please anyone, including himself. That makes things much worse in his life because he has to be dependent on other people and that can really hurt a person.Ask yourself two questions. First, the activity that you are doing now or contemplating doing now, will it bring forth reward this week or will it drain time, energy, money, or effort? The second question: if you were going to die next week, would it matter? You could stand in front of a mirror and look at yourself, see if you are happy with yourself the way you are right now. If you are, then continue what you are doing, but if not then you need to change a few things.

Realize that the only way you are going to change anything is by committing and setting up your priorities. Many people set resolutions only to fail at them within a couple of weeks because they set themselves up to do so. When you decide upon an action, you must completely commit to it, or else why bother with the attempt at all?

You must also set your boundaries. If you do not leave your job back at the office, if you bring it with you wherever you go, twenty-four hours a day, then you are never going to find the time to improve yourself. The first important rule, then, is to set aside time for just yourself and family. Leave your work at work, and allow yourself personal time in the home. This principle is very important!

Similarly, for your health if you have allotted time for exercising or whatever you plan to encourage health, then do not to let the stress of your job encroach upon that time. Commit to your health and set the boundaries between time for that and the other aspects of your life.

2. Good Breathing

The majority of people do not know how to breathe. They breathe too shallow, are stressed out, and are constantly in the old fight-or-flight mode. Well, that was great when we fought lions and tigers and had to beat off things to live, but it is only a survival mechanism and not necessary for our current day-to-day living. You really need to get to a place where you can understand who you are and become one with yourself, with nature, and with God. Breathing is one of the most powerful mechanisms by which to do this, but too many of us just do not know how to breathe. They breathe shallow, losing about 20% of the oxygen that should be getting to their lungs, which results in an increase in the risk of all kinds of malignancies as well as in free radical damage, which in turn promotes inflammation. It is a vicious cycle, so the number one exercise you can do is to learn how to breathe properly.

When you breathe from the diaphragm or abdomen, you use muscles that you have not used before because you are usually using your neck and chest muscles to breathe shallow. Babies breathe from the abdomen because this is how God created us to breathe. Abdominal breathing takes the stress off the neck and chest, reducing headaches and TMJ (Temporomandibular *Joint Dysfunction*). Your sinuses will also improve.

Alternate nasal breathing is one method I recommend. Close one nostril with your finger, then breathe in through the open one to a count of 4, hold your breath for about 7 seconds, then slowly breathe out to a count of 8. While breathing out, hold your tongue up to the roof of your mouth to create a whooshing sound over that 8-count. Then switch nostrils.

I also use imaging with the breathing. Breathe in a white light (I usually call it God's light or something similar), and while breathing, imagine that you are breathing in the healing manifestation and breathing out all of your frustration and stress. Let your body go with this exercise, forget the past and never mind about the future. Because one of the most beneficial things about breathing is it gets you directly into the present.

The key benefit physically is your Cortisol level. The Cortisol level indicates that stress is highest at eight o'clock in the morning. That is why most of the time people have heart attacks in the morning as they are going off to work on a Monday. A high Cortisol level means higher stress and hence higher risk of heart attacks and other stress related disorders. You are waking up from essentially an almost death-like state called sleep repair, and then you have to get going! After that, your Cortisol level drops off as the day goes on. You might spike a little with events of the day, then around 5 or 6 in the evening you have an even higher spike, though not as great as in the morning. This is when I recommend doing all these exercises mentioned. It is when the cortisol is the highest. High cortisol promotes high glucose levels and low insulin levels, which is a toxic combination. Overtime this unregulated high cortisol will produce cells that are not responsive to the uptake of glucose (insulin resistance). It is like one time when I was in North Carolina in a paper mill town and I asked the locals how they could stand the smell. They asked me, "what smell?" They had been there for so long that they could not even smell the odor due to accommodation. It still did not mean that there were no consequences of the toxic fumes. The sugar problem is just an adjustment that the body makes to prolong life when we do not maintain good lifestyles.

The issue is to promote a lower blood sugar level to balance the sympathetic nervous system. Shift it from a fight or flight mode into a relaxation phase that will allow you to process the sugar and get it out of your system. An important part of doing this is to improve the oxygenation, and the best time to do that is in the morning. During the day, you get busy with work, appointments, errands, and what not, and you forget you need to breathe properly. In the morning, though, about an hour before eating, you have this quiet period of time when you can get back to yourself and shift your metabolism in a tremendous way to promote healing, regeneration, and the energy you will have for the day. You do not have to run for coffee or anything else to get stimulated. You are already stimulated because you have allowed your body to go to a different place in your life. Learning how to breathe properly is incredibly important.

Another technique I use is a CD that has the frequencies of oxygen, nitrogen, hydrogen, and the central elements playing. Just listen to these frequencies while you are breathing in this complete state of relaxation and it promotes more lymphatic activation that cleans out the body's toxins. Just doing this will increase your oxygenation tremendously as well as keeping your heart healthy.

Wherever you choose to do the breathing exercise, just make sure it is in a quiet place, away from cell phones, pagers, and noisy distractions.

3. Visualization

I frequently do guided visualization with people, teaching them visualization skills as well. When you look at visualization, you are looking at a part of the brain that humans use not very often. A part that we are unaware that we use, but we use it all the time. This part is the neocortex and the thalamus.

Here is a checklist to help you with visualization: The environment is very important; a quiet place that is free from all the affairs of the day, where you can get into the Present. Do some breathing exercises and progressive relaxation; start from the bottom of your feet, going slowly up to the top of your head, flexing and relaxing your muscles as you go, visualizing that you are in an elevator going to the top. Breathing will quieten your mind and attention to you alone, which is the most important thing you can possibly do because you are the most important thing in your life.

When you begin visualizing activities you want to do, the crazier it is (the more shapes and colors involved), the better it is. I call this the hilarity factor. The body responds to pictures and images, as does the heart. The body has memory in the brain, so too does the heart have its own memory. What you want to do is imprint this enough on your heart, which allows for the freeing of the brain so it can do the healing that the body needs. It is important to create a visual impression that promotes health and wellness. If you can shock it by imagining something foolish then that is great.

For example, if you have a colon issue, you could imagine a tiny man with a clothespin on his nose, inside your colon with a broom vigorously sweeping out the trash and rotten debris. The more disastrous a condition someone has, the better results the person will have with visualization.

If you have abnormal cells in your body, then the typical thing is to picture Pac-man as your immune system. Little blue Pac-man, coming through and gobbling up these bad cells and debris, frowning at first until he gobbles up a few abnormal cells then gets this bright smile on his face, and even turns a brighter shade of blue. How much do you need to do this? Just enough to fake the brain into believing that it is helping eliminate the abnormal cells. You need to get the brain and the heart to believe that this is actually going on instead of the gloom and doom the doctor told you to believe.

The key to this is getting to the level where the brain and heart work together, which is down in the delta or theta realms of brain wave activity. Delta and Theta brain waves occur within the first couple of hours of initiating sleep and are slow waves. These waves allow the body to heal so it is important to go to bed early or you just might miss your healing. I have ways of helping people get to those levels while awake and they can have miraculous results. REM (Rapid Eye Movement) sleep is the time you do most of your dreaming and it allows one to consolidate the memories of the day. This allows for the creation of strong visual images that become your reality.

Our thoughts have much power to create, so we have to be careful about what we are thinking, lest we create that which we did not intend. Avoid thoughts or images that bring you down all the time, because it is very important that you visualize that which is the best and how it is good for your body at that time.

Visualization is a great way of getting into the Present, allowing your body to realize there is an alternative pattern. Just imagining that the possibility could exist is all it takes; the body will run with it and create some absolutely incredible results. Thoughts are multi-dimensional holographic pictures that are stored in the cellular memory of the heart. The heart, when operating out of fear, is constantly checking the senses and the emotions that the neurons wire together and seeing if there is a match from the past. It is like a library of our thoughts and if it finds a match, it will pull it up and we will re-live it. I had an 11-year-old young man tell me a secret about my iPhone. The programs I was running depleted my battery every night and I had to recharge it so I asked him to help me solve the mystery. He told me to see what was running in the background. I said, "What's the background?" I had 85 programs running that I no longer needed so I quickly removed them and now my battery is working fine. How many old beliefs are running in the background on your heart's hard drive that you no longer need? Remember, thoughts originate from the heart and thoughts put to action is emotion that is based on our belief systems or better known as the color of glasses we wear, our perceptions. If we change our "stinking" thinking, we can change our beliefs and change our lives.

4. Grounding

Grounding is something that is completely free. All you have to do is walk outside on your bare feet. The earth has electromagnetic fields and so do we. We are like a battery, with a positive and a negative charge. The earth and everything on it has its own polarity, so when lightning strikes the earth it energizes it with electrons, giving it the negative charge that it typically has.

We have high levels of free radical damage that goes on over time and this free radical damage brings positive charge or acidity into the body. This damage can come from such things as heavy metal toxicity, pollutants of all kinds, cell phones, any source of electromagnetic radiation around our lives causing a lot of destruction, especially the carrier wave on which the data our phone transmits information.

The phone experts do not test the carrier wave-induced damage. This is a problem, but standard medical practice says everything is all right, but these frequencies actually interfere with the human body. They build up acidity, the result of too many positive charges. We need to discharge these, and the best way is to connect to the earth. When we wear rubber sole shoes, plastics, and things that insolate us from the earth, we build up this problem of positive potential.

Things that are associated with inflammation become an issue; the autoimmune diseases, diabetes, gout, lupus, rheumatoid arthritis, carpal tunnel syndrome, cardiovascular disease, all forms of malignancies. These are all associated with increased inflammation in the body. The earth itself, though, is a great antioxidant.

As described in The Most Important Health Discovery Ever by Basic Health Publications, Inc., physicists and electrical engineers have chosen the Earth as the most obvious "ground," or reference point, for all electrical power grids. The Earth provides a reference voltage, that is, the ground or zero potential against which all other voltages are established and measured. What is measured is the difference in electric potential between two points, one being the Earth. The second reference point is the body. Being grounded means your body's internal organs are shielded from any electrostatic or electromagnetic interference in the atmosphere. This provides for a very quiet electrical 'milieu' inside the body where no external electric or magnetic fields can disrupt the internal functions maintaining homeostasis and health. This is very important; we have the responsibility to maintain this balance in our bodies. These functions include digestion, internal repairs, wound healing, and all metabolic activities. Keep in mind that all chemical or biochemical reactions are electrical in nature and so are susceptible to being disturbed by external electric and magnetic fields. Grounding prevents these disturbances.

All people need to do is just get out onto a good plot of grass or hold onto a tree. Just be careful of grass grown with pesticides and electrical wires under the ground. What happens is a current flow starts, between you and the earth. Electrons in the earth feed up into your body, reducing your positive charge...like hot air moving into cold air, filling in a deficiency.

There are also devices that you can connect to walls, in the ground, or even run outside through a window and into the ground. One has a silver sheet inside of the lining that improves the conductivity between you and the ground. Afterwards you can see the improvement in your heart rate variability and oxygen saturation. For years prior to grounding, I could not improve my coherency and heart rate variability higher than average challenge. I decided to see what grounding was doing for me so I initially did the heart rate variability study first and then did it grounded only for 5 min, and I saw it improve by 80%. Within days, I was up to the 3 and 4 highest challenge level. I was convinced, even though I initially did not think it was doing anything. I now recommend grounding for everyone.

The electrons that are predominant in the earth move into a place that has a lower number of electrons, so it is like a nutrient. I consider the earth as a nutrient. The electrons go in there, remove the free radicals, then come out the other side and down into the ground. It is a natural exchange going on at all times that improves your blood viscosity, which is essential for good cardiac health. Studies prove if the blood is too thick and toxic, heart attacks and strokes incidence increase. Looking under a microscope, you will see red blood cells that are stuck together, but in just a matter of minutes of contact with the earth, an increase in oxygenation and thinning of the blood occurs. The blood becomes more free flowing and less able to block the circulatory system.

The place for your grounding is, of course, outside and the best time is at night. The body performs the bulk of its healing between 11pm and 5am. An optimal time for grounding would be while you sleep. However, this is not an option for most people, so do it at a time that works for you. Grounding is good any time you want to do it. Just kick off your shoes, walk around, daydream, read, write, garden, whatever. You will reduce inflammation, improve your longevity, and get more benefit than drugs could ever offer.

5. Laughing

Laughter is also free and it is very healthy. It is true that laughter is the best medicine. It improves the immune system by 40%, and oxygenation increases from the gulping of air that you do while laughing. Just 10 minutes of laughing is all it takes. There are all sorts of reports of medical miracles brought about by laughter. One example is the Stage III Cancer patient who watched comedy movies for a month and went into remission.

There are 15 different facial muscles involved in laughing that you would not otherwise use. The act of laughing improves oxygenation in the body, and balances hormone levels, such as from the adrenal glands or serotonin. Just a few minutes of daily laughter is enough to show improvement. You will also burn about 50 calories, and any burning of calories is a good thing. Laughter is also good for relieving stress and anxiety, increasing dopamine, and increasing the production of a little molecule named Cytokine. This molecule activates the immune system's front line warrior cells and from there revs up all aspects of your immune system from the mucus in your nasal passages to your intestinal tract.

Laughter is also very contagious, so if you hear someone laughing then find a way to get closer. You can make a new friend and get healthier all at the same time! Laughter puts you in the Present, removes your stress and anxieties, and makes it impossible to be upset.

I recommend laughing at least twice a day for at least 10 minutes if possible. The variety of laughing is also important, because you do not want to get bored with one type of laugh. So laugh high, laugh low, laugh in between; laugh fast, laugh slow, laugh about life, laugh about yourself, but just start laughing. If you have somebody around, they will be laughing with you and will not even have a clue about what you are laughing. When you are incredibly stressed out or worried about something, thinking of something funny is the *last* thing on your mind, but that is when you need laughter the most. It will put you in a far better place to deal with the troubles in your life. Start the day off with a laugh, laugh about an hour before eating, and your day will go a whole lot better. Try to combine laughing and the breathing exercises. They are a tremendous combination.

6. Walking

The best way to walk is barefoot, because it improves the posture of the body and the contour of your spine. The body is not designed to protect itself when you are in a hard shoe, when there is no flexibility, so the best thing is to either walk barefoot (just be careful about where you step or what you step in) or walk with flexible shoes. Hard shoes are bad for posture, plus you need to get a spring off your back feet when walking. I do not recommend running because running is traumatic to the joints, particularly in females. When you run you have a lower center of gravity, it puts more stress on the structures and the body. Fast walking is fine, but not running.

Swimming, of course, is another way people can safely exercise, but you need to make sure the pool is chlorine free, because that could be worse than not doing anything at all. You can find a salt-water pool or one that works through ionic means. Oh and make sure you walk to and from the pool... if it is not too far!

Do not take great strides when you walk. This type of walking throw your body out of balance and increase the risk of straining. Walk with a normal stride, or simply walk faster. A foot and a half or two is fine, depending on how tall you are. Throwing your hands far out and back just wastes too much energy and does not get you anywhere faster, not to mention it creates a drag on your body. I recommend having your arms at 90 degrees and alternating them, which is the natural progression of walking in the first place, so it is not really anything you need to focus on. Just do it and get your heart rate up. Go slow at first, don't bite off more than you can chew; start off with 10 to 15 minutes, and do it outside where there is a lesser concentration of toxins. An aerated environment is always best.

Walking should never be a stressful thing, but something you enjoy. It is a great pain killer, increases endorphins, clears your mind and helps you focus. Walk with someone you enjoy walking with, because walking alone could increase the likelihood that you could lose the habit. Walk with someone who can push you, someone you can have a friendly competition. Alternatively, take along a pet dog…or a child. Both have boundless energy that forces you to keep up!

7. Eating

Eating is another very important aspect of health, wellbeing and longevity. Where, when, how, and what to eat all are associated into getting the most out of your food. I will not get into the wide range of diets, but will just cover some general rules about eating. It is very important to talk about eating, because it is another method of coming into the Present.

When I talk with my patients about eating, when I discuss diet, we always have a B.L.A.S.T. The reason that people eat so much is because they are Bored, Lonely, Angry, Sad or Tired. I tell people that near the dinner table, on the refrigerator, and in their billfold or purse, they should have this acronym. When they have the desire to eat unhealthy food they should determine the risk and benefit by engaging their rational reasoning of the left prefrontal cortex by having this posted somewhere so they can see it prior to eating.

You are in a good sympathetic tone when in a state of relaxation, so you should always eat in a relaxed setting. Never eat when you are stressed; take your time to eat, chew thoroughly, relax. The digestive process actually begins with the first smell, with the initial intention to eat. Then when you put the food in your mouth, the digestive juices are ready, and you need to chew thoroughly until it is essentially in a liquefied form that you can swallow. Just the simple act of chewing completely reduces much of the acid reflux that goes on today, because when an undigested lump hits the stomach, it has to create that additional acidity to digest it. The key, then, is to eat in a way that is comfortable, relaxed, and at a slow pace.

Perhaps you have heard the old saying "eat to live, live to eat". Most people just live to eat and they end up very sick because they do not do the most critical thing, which is to enjoy their food, to savor their food, to get as many senses involved as possible when they are actually eating. People allow their fork to be a weapon of mass destruction. In my home state of Mississippi, we have the highest level of obesity in the nation. 60% of our people are overweight and 40% of those are considered obese. This is, in large part, due to a "give me" mentality. People do not want to take responsibility and they rely on others for too many of their solutions in life.

The other thing that is really important is our food choices. Not only do our bodies have an electromagnetic charge, but our food has a positive or negative charge as well. We call this spin activity. Positive spin activity means it spins to the right, negative spin means it spins to the left. We need to eat food that has a right spin (clockwise), for the same reason that it benefits us to walk barefoot on the negatively charged earth. Clockwise spin usually comes from naturally produced food. The following figure should illustrate this concept.

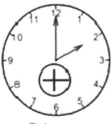

D-Isomer

Usually occurs naturally.

Healthy

Firewood for example.

Builds up the body.

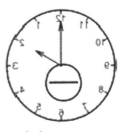

L-Isomer

Usually synthetic.

Unhealthy.

Microwave for example.

Breaks down body.

If you look at Vitamin E, for instance, you will see that it says Alpha D-tocopherol; that "D" means it is from a natural source. If you see an "L" instead, then that means it is from a synthetic source; it has some Vitamin D in it. Of course the Alpha-tocopherol is not the most important anyway, the Gamma is. Many so-called nutrition companies, though, will not give you the really essential nutrients because they want to do whatever it takes to maximize their profits. The products they sell are most of the time absolute junk. They leave out all the good things and add in all the bad, which gives it a negative spin, promoting destruction of the body instead of building it up. One example of this is any kind of genetically modified food. Grains, for instance, stay away from grains.

I like to start people off with a basic diet. Ninety percent of the population has some form of gluten sensitivity, so if I can get them off wheat, oats, barley, and rye, all those glutens that are gluing up their gastrointestinal tracts and interfering with absorption, then within two weeks they feel like a miracle has taken place in their bodies. They can then put things in their diet that can promote health instead of sickness and degeneration, and reduce the inflammation. Probably the best test you can do to see if you are gluten sensitive is simply stay off it for a while, stay away from dairy, and see how you feel after a few weeks.

Avoid soy at all cost, because soy is one of those left spin foods. It interferes with the body's ability to properly process hormones and can cause some severe issues in the body. Fermented soy is okay and it may also have some benefits associated with it, but the food produces genetically modifies our soy in the United States. When you genetically modify something, it is artificial, has no life force in it, and causes many issues.

Another thing is high fructose corn syrup. One of the worst things a person can put in their body is this sugar substitute. It looks like sucrose, which is sugar as far as the composition between fructose and the glucose molecule, but the problem is that it really does not create an insulin spike. The body needs that insulin spike to tell it that we are getting full and need to shut down the hunger and eating process. High fructose corn syrup will allow an increase in Ghrelin, which is a hormone that tells a body to crave calories; this is a contributing factor with becoming very overweight.

That is not to say that artificial sweeteners are any better because they are far worse. They all have very dangerous agents that prompt the body to attack itself. One study done at the Health Science Center in Texas compared regular sugar drinks with artificial sweetener drinks and showed an over 60% increased risk of obesity for using artificial sweeteners compared to the regular sugar drinks in general. Consequently, I definitely do not recommend any sugar drinks at all. Just stick with good clean water; it will improve oxygenation to the cell and more ably cleanse the body.

When should I eat?

The best time to eat is around 8am when your cortisol level is the highest, and 10am when the cortisol level drops down and it is time for a little snack. Apple, nuts, green shake, and organic yogurts could be an option if you are not allergic or sensitive to dairy. I would avoid free fructose but apples eaten in their natural state have fiber and other balancing agents. Fructose, and the fruit juices they come in, is very important to avoid. All fruit is good, but you need to stay away from the higher Glycemic sugars such as bananas, cantaloupes and watermelons. Indulge your-self in cherries, blueberries, raspberries, and all those wonderful berries. Another wonderful quote from Dr. Bruce Bond is when people ask what is a carbohydrate? His answer is if it has no father or mother, if it does not sink or swim, it is a carbohydrate. The greatest threat to America today is the excessive carbohydrates which lowers the Growth Hormone and pro-motes obesitis (inflammation of the fat cells.)

The best time to eat fruit is in the morning, prior to your exercise routine, and separate from breakfast. You should do your exercising about an hour before eating breakfast. Avoid drinking any water while eating; if you do, drink lukewarm water and very little, because water re-ally impairs the digestive system.

Eat lunch around 12 or 1pm, then a light snack later on when Corti-sol levels fall and you need to stabilize your blood sugar. It is better for you to save the carbohydrates for the evening: starches, beans that type meal. Evening meals should be the lightest meal of the day, because you have to get ready for digestion through the night. If you are going to eat meat, you should eat the meat at lunch.

You always want to do your exercising about an hour before eating. I recommend a pinch of Himalayan sea salt with an 8 oz glass of water prior to exercising, as well as one hour before and after meals. Try to drink half your body weight in ounces of pure clean water throughout the day. Keep your meals free of any water or fluid ingestion of any kind.

Another issue I have difficulties with is the alkaline water systems that people use. The body's blood pH is controlled at a very steady value of around 7.4-7.5; too much and you die, too little and you die. The body is all about balance and you have two high tides and two low tides per day, just like the ocean. The first thing I do with a patient is to do a weekly food diary and look and see what is missing or excessive in their diet. Another incentive is to check your pH at 8am prior to breakfast, 1pm prior to lunch, 6pm prior to dinner, and 8pm 2 hours after your last meal. You should measure your pH using your saliva and urine, and it should be above 6.5 half of the time and less than 6.5 the other half.

Promotion of tumor can occur in an alkaline environment and some tumors grow in an acid environment. We have to determine whether a person is anabolic or catabolic. I have seen so many people come in drinking alkaline water for 6 months and then found out they have cancer. Now I cringe when I hear alkaline water! The stomach also requires acidity to properly digest food and over 50% of the population has low stomach acid. Many medications require acidity to work. So one must be careful when they use alkaline water, and they first need an evaluation of a trained professional.

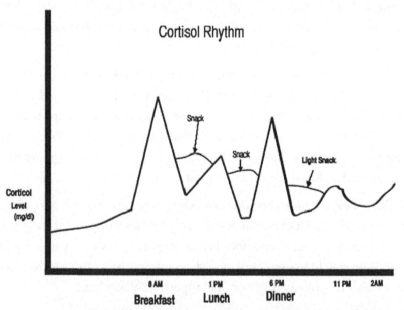

Recommendation is to lower cortisol by meditation and exercise one hour before eating breakfast and dinner, around 7Am and 5PM.
The purpose is to smooth out the curve and increase dopamine and serotonin which help with awarding and depressive symtoms.

If you are on any sort of medication, you need to consult with your physician before following this regimen. There can be some very serious issues with medications and interference from what you eat.

Eat well. Eat with people you enjoy. Dr. Bruce Bond says *"your body is a temple not an outhouse."* You must treat it that way. Eating is supposed to be the most enjoyable thing. Avoid eating with people that will stress you out, and people who are snobs or those who cause ruckus.

Eating should be a very enjoyable thing. Most importantly, pray before you eat. Bless your food and appreciate it for what it is doing to promote life.

These are the seven different activities that you can do to promote thinking that is more responsible and a life that is healthier and longer. You can perform many of them together, so not having the time is not a valid excuse for not doing them. These are very simple solutions. They can also save you money in the end because you are not wasting money on a bunch of junk! You will also avoid having to suffer the financial expense incurred from sickness and disease. You get a payoff with the rewards of health and wellness. If you did nothing else but these simple steps, you could improve your health by more than 50%.

All you have to do is simply be there for your body.

The Case Of Tammy Holt

At the age of 36, I had heart problems in the form of a severe heart arrhythmia, mental stress, and bad migraines over a period of 2 to 3 weeks, finally culminating in one migraine for 2 days nonstop.

I saw the appropriate doctors, and they found my heart was close to the size of a basketball, with 25% usage, and they gave me 2 to 3 years to live. I was given medications for both my heart and the migraines, including Lasix, Coreg, Lisinopril, and Maxalt. But nothing helped.

My mom had used Dr. Lucky before, so I decided to give him a try. He took me off the Maxalt, put me on a special diet, and gave me some natural supplements and vitamins to take, as well as some light-energized water.

He then went over my life to find what problems in my head might be affecting my body. He discovered that a physical problem I had every 7 years was due to a past bad relationship with a man, and also discovered the issues I had with my father. He then brought out a heart-shaped stone that was already broken and said it symbolized my relationship with my father, and then told me to bury it in a place where I felt happiest. My father had been doing the best that he knew how and it was now time to forgive him; he prayed with me as I buried it. Dr. Lucky then gave me a list of self- affirmations to tell myself every day.

Within days my problems began to clear away. One month later I had no more migraines, I had more energy, and, after a year, my heart rhythm was back to normal and up to 50% usage. The heart doctors could not believe it when they saw a more normal sized heart. They said that only rarely would the rhythmic problem I had convert back to normal.

It is amazing, the way he helped me! What he is doing really works!

The Doctor's Notes:

Thirty-six year young white female who had severe heart arrhythmia for about 6 years and the cardiologist had told her she would have to live with the condition, and one doctor even told her that it did not matter about her diet or if she exercised. They told her 4 years ago she would be dead in two to three years because of her severely dilated, thin walled heart. Her echocardiogram indicated an EF% (Ejection Fraction of the Heart) in the 20's, with normal around 50 to 60. The doctor prescribed to her Coreg, Lasix, and Lisinopril, and her EF improved to around 30 but her rhythm never changed. She came to my office for severe headaches lasting four weeks for which she was taking Maxalt, without much help. She had to sleep about every two hours and had significant lower extremity edema. She had a significant issue with her weight on exam, O2 sats (oxygen saturation) low for a person her age at 96% on room air. She had quite irregular heartbeat about every 3 beats and possibly s3 gallop (third heart sound) indicating heart failure, her PMI (point of maximum impulse) was weak and very lateral. She was having a short run of SVT (Supraventricular Tachycardia) for 3 beats, then a regular beat, followed by PVC (Premature Ventricular Tachycardia) in a repeating sequence. I knew this was dangerous, but she told me this was normal for her.

We discontinued her Maxalt and told her if her fluid got better, we will have to reduce the lasix.

We recommended low grain diet, avoidance of all sugar synthetically altered, and placed her on vitamin B's, omega three, vitamin D, coenzyme Q10, proteolytic enzymes, taurine, and glyconutrients. We used a crystal in the shape of a heart that was already broken to symbolize her relationship to her father for burial and discussed forgiveness and the idea that her father was doing the best he knew. She allowed us to pray with her and we released her home.

1 month later she had much better energy, the headaches had all but disappeared, she no longer had to sleep every two hours, edema was much better at a 3+ to 1+ grading of the swelling of her legs, and her heart

would beat 8 times without irregularities. She had not changed her diet. We discussed her amazing improvement; you could hardly recognize her from the first visit.

The big surprise happened several months ago when she saw the Cardiologist and the cardiologist checked her pulse and said something was wrong. He then ordered an EKG followed by an ECHO. Then he shook his head in disbelief, because she was in normal rhythm and her ECHO was now 50%. The doctor told her the rhythm she had rarely converted back to normal.

She then called my office and left a message thanking Jesus, thanking Dr. Lucky, thanking Jesus, thanking Dr. Lucky, thanking Jesus, thanking Dr. Lucky…You get the idea. I believe she should thank Jesus and thank herself for taking control of her health. Her diet is much better and she now has something to live for. She has hope.

The Case Of Marie Bridget Vicknair Stephens

I had generally terrible health. I was rundown, bloated, swollen, and mentally exhausted. My daughter had used Dr. Lucky for two years, so I went to see him. He had me fill out a questionnaire about my family and siblings, and then proceeded to diagnose me by just by looking at me, without any tests that traditional medical doctors would give. As seems usual for the rest of his patients, my first visit was a long one; about four hours.

I had been taking quite a large range of supplements, so he cut them down to only those absolutely necessary. Then he found that I had emotional issues; I had my first child when I was 15, and that created an anxiety that I was still feeling, as well as other family and friends issues. Just by dealing with these problems, my health improved dramatically.

I had weight issues, and surgery for it about 12 years ago, but Dr. Lucky said that I was just gluten intolerant, which fit with the fact that I had eaten 100% wheat for 10 years. I dropped gluten from my diet and dropped 9 pounds in the first month, 6 pounds the next.

I had a bump on my arm that Dr. Lucky found without touching. He put a mustard patch on the bump, concentrated, then within minutes the bump was gone.

He also had me meditate to help me relax. Before I went into his office I couldn't lift both hands above my head. Now it is not a problem. I continue with the meditation. It cleanses my body and soul and keeps my mind alert.

Within 3 months' time, I went from 65 years old to a vibrant me-maw.

When I first saw Dr. Lucky, I did not know how to feel in his presence. I know now it was the Holy Spirit in him, mending my soul and mind. He is way ahead of his field and I recommend him to anyone to heal their heart, mind, and body. He is a very Godly man.

The Doctor's Notes:

A wonderful Christian lady that had recently seen me so I wanted to include her in my book. We have not done any follow up lab but I just love her and her wonderful daughter. I really cannot take credit for what has happened in her life and her family's life.

I had found the lump during a scan without touching. She said she had noticed it was sore for quite a while.

" *For bodily exercise profiteth little:
but godliness is profitable unto all things,
having promise of the life that now is, and
of that which is to come.* "

I Timothy 4:8 KJV Holy Bible

Chapter THREE

7 Strategies To Exercise Your Mind & Body

Men throughout the ages protected and provided for their families. When you are out in the woods and see a roaring lion, there is no time to react emotionally, no time to see, no time to play music to the lion or draw a painting of it. It is either fight or flight. Thus, according to the American Psychological Association, the left-brain knows what the right brain is doing. (Michael Price, January of 2009, volume 40, number 1, page 60). 90% of the population is right handed and 95% of these righties are in their left cerebral cortex. But only about 20% of the lefties actually have that laterality, and so that 20% divide the duties not so originally involved. Society favors the left-brain behavior.In school, we learn to read the English language left to right, and this is all in a left-brain pattern that focuses on being analytical, sequential, and linear thinkers, instead of creative thinkers and doing creative mathematics. We focus more on conformity and the lack of change instead of breaking the rules and society's norms. Notice the languages that read in the opposite direction from English: Chinese, Japanese, Arabic, and Hebrew. They all read right to left and they are the leading economic people today. Why is this? Because their brains are in a creative atmosphere, whereas our English reader friends are actually decreasing in proficiency. Therefore, the question is… what determines normal?

The Magnesium levels of a particular patient concerned me, because I found out the level had changed significantly from 1.6 to 1.8 then back to 1.6, so I called the lab to see what was going on. They told me that they had a change and 1.6mg/dl was now normal, so I said, *"Well, what deter-mines normal?"* They replied, *"What we do is draw blood on the people in the lab and come up with the mean, then we take that measurement and we make two standard deviations on each side and that's how we come up with our normals"*. I then said, *"Well, you know something? I have patients that are really feeling unhealthy and are definitely not normal yet they have a Magne-sium level of 1.6. They need Magnesium."*

It really depends on what determines normal.

We also look at the average body and observe that it is extremely nu-tritionally deficient. This is due in large part to obesity, especially in the state of Mississippi where about 60% of the people are overweight and unhealthy. Those same studies, however, also indicate that many schizo-phrenics are left-handers. In some nations overseas, a large percentage of the population would be considered schizophrenic. Yet these are some of the most creative people around. Our jail system is also loaded with peo-ple just not understood. It is all about who makes the rules and sets the standards.

We know that most people do not get enough exercise. The most exercise they get is handling the remote control on TV, or texting nonstop on cell phones, or playing video games. Recently the Ameri-can Medical Association released a study saying that the linkage of watching television two to three hours a day or more increases the risk of diabetes, cardiovascular disease, and early death from all causes. The big issue today in most people's minds is that we are not exercising our left-brain enough. But the bigger issue is that we are not exercising our right brain, tapping into our creative side and get-ting out there and *doing* something, figuring out more creative ways of getting healthier.

When I first see a male patient walk into my clinic, I get a bit con-cerned, so I have a special test that I do with him called the paper clip test. I tell him to write down in 2 minutes how many things that one can do with a paper clip. The majority of men get about 3 to 4, whereas women get about 9 to 10. If the man actually does pretty well, because his mind just goes on and on, then great. But if he has a low score, then I know my work is cut out for the day, because I am going to have a hard time breaking that mindset.

Typically, a man believes in facts and figures (even though stats are often untrustworthy). Their reliance on data causes them to be skeptical and restrained. I see this skepticism play out in my male to female patient ratio. About 95% of the people whom I treat are women. Of the remaining 5%, 2.5 percent are men that their wives or mother brings in and they are only coming to an appointment with me to prove that I am crazy and what I am doing is actually wrong. Another 1% of the men are lefties, so they are more open because they are using their right brains. Then the remaining 1.5 percent of the men come to me because they actually want to prolong life and get healthy. These men are genuinely looking for healthier alternatives in life.

America has an epidemic of left-brain thinkers and one of the focuses of this book is to introduce the musical, the artistic, the humorous, the creative nonconformist spontaneous side of life to America. As such, I will begin with mental exercises designed to wake up the other half of your brain, then later filter in some physical exercises that you can do to improve your health. Even in the Bible, it states that bodily exercise can profit a little, but that exercising your brain can profit much. The ideal, then, is a combination of the two, and it is with a couple examples of these that we shall start.

The Cross Crawl

The first technique to help balance the left and right brain is an exercise called the cross crawl. While standing, lift and bend your left leg and swing over with the right hand, then pat your left knee. Then alternate beginning with the right leg. Do this in the morning for about two minutes, before you eat your breakfast, to get your circulation going. As I said in the previous chapter, you need to lower your Cortisol level, reduce insulin resistance, and prepare your body for eating to speed up your metabolism. This process also allows you to clear your mind and get ready for your day. Thus, a cross crawl is both a physical and a mental exercise. If you are physically unable to do the exercise, an alternative is to sit in a chair rather than on the floor. If you are still unable to do the exercise, then you can just imagine lifting up your legs and crossing your arms. Your intent is what matters.

Alternate Nasal Breathing

The second exercise that works both physical and mental is alternate nasal breathing. It is an aerobic technique that originated in India known there as Panayama. I use this technique quite often, and is relaxing to myself. It allows you to get into the Present Moment. I recommend the cross crawl just to get things started, then you can sit down in a nice confusion-free spot, turn off cell phones and other noise-makers, and breathe. We know the right-brain controls the left nostril and the left-brain controls the right nostril, and this is very important.

When we talk about the right nostril and the left-brain, we are talking about the linear, the sequential, and the mathematical. The left-brain also has fewer alpha waves that are involved with meditation and deeper levels of brain activity that bring you into the Present. You focus your concern on the environment, whether something is chasing you, or if you are hungry and need to get your food. On the opposite side, the left nostril controls the right brain, where everything is calm and relaxed, so this is the focal area when you go to bed at night; you are digesting, respiratory and heart rate falls, all those wonderful things that have to do with relaxation and creativity. Imagination actually improves in this situation.

Your nose clogs up about every 2 hours, but it does so unequally; a free nasal passage indicates the half of the brain more open to activity. As a result, there are times when you are more open to logical thinking and others when you are more creative. This breathing exercise, then, allows you to work both sides of the brain at the same time, and as a bonus, it is also good for your respiratory system.

You start by placing a finger on the outside of the left side of your nose to close your left nostril, leaving the right nostril is open. Breathe in deeply through the right nostril for about 4 seconds, then hold your breath about 2 seconds, then exhale for 4 seconds. Then switch nostrils, holding the right side closed, breathe in through the left and repeat the pattern. Repeat this several times, alternately breathing through one nostril then the other.

This will put you more into the Present, and activate the more creative right side of the brain, putting you more in balance. It will also help improve sleep, calm emotions, improve your digestion, and boost your memory and thinking power. It is also good for those who suffer with insomnia. Just close your right nostril and breathe through the left; this activates the right brain and increases the parasympathetic nervous system that helps you to sleep.

Those two exercises help you both mentally and physically. Now let us look first at seven exercises for improved mental activity.

1. Brain Storming

Everyone knows about brainstorming. Big companies do it to get an upper hand on the competition. It is simply free association. It is the opposite of constrained thinking. You have people of different beliefs and thought patterns, right and left-brain thinkers together. They are eclectic mix of thinkers who initiate ideas that at first do not even make sense. The ideas get increasingly specific and you end up with the final product. The group generally does brainstorming collectively, but it can be done alone as well. Just start free associating, doodle or draw graphs, whatever it takes to shake the ideas loose. Brainstorming is about spontaneity.

2. Mind Mapping

I have done a tremendous amount of mind mapping. It begins when you come up with an idea, and then combine it with brainstorming. The nervous system is its own microcosm, greatly resembling a tree. You have the main trunk of the cell body, called the soma, and from this projects the branches, called dendrites that allow for communication between the neurons. These connections join in a myriad of ways, meeting at what scientists call the axon where the nervous conductivity takes place. Electrical impulses cross a gap called a synapse to other neurons. You have about 10 billion of these in the average brain, all connected in what looks very much like a tree. You start out with a main idea and then you have all these branches coming off, and this is what a mind map represents. Each one of these 10 billion neurons in the human brain has a possible number of connections equal to a 1 followed by 28 zeros, so one can hardly imagine what the entire brain is capable of. The number of possible combinations in the brain, if written out, would be 1 followed by 10.5 million kilometers of zeros, so you know we're not even scratching the surface of what we can do. This data comes from the Mind Map Book from Barry Buzan, a guru in mind mapping.

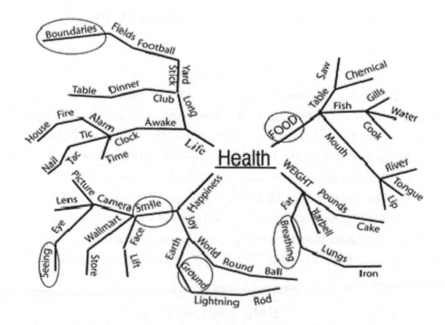

When I perform mind mapping, I start with a graph, divided up into three areas representing Mind, Body, and Spirit. The individual starts out with the mind, drawing a picture of a brain, for instance, and any thought that comes to mind that has to do with…the mind. Then color it in; I recommend having all kinds of colors because that helps to activate the right side of the brain. If your next thought is a light bulb for an idea, then color one in.

If your next thought is an emotion, then draw that emotion. If you are sad, then draw a sad face in the Spirit part of the graph. If you are thinking about something to do with your body, like a leg injury for example, then draw that in the Body part of the graph. Continue this way with free association, drawing different things into the different branches until the whole of them come to mean something to you. Until you find a commonality within them.

For example, you could draw fire in the Brain section, because fire needs oxygen to fuel it, to keep it burning bright. You may draw an angel for the Spirit to represent how God figures into your life. For the Body, you might draw a heart, or someone on a bicycle, or someone swimming, etc. This exercise has the potential to generate a tremendous amount of information and can create incredible ideas.

3. Design A Funny File

I have said that laughter is important, particularly for a stressed out person, because he lacks stress if he is laughing. Take anything you find amusing, whether it be from joke books, cartoons, humorous news items, funny looking objects, and then put them into a file. This will be your treasure chest to open in times of sorrow and stress, something to lift you up from depression or relieve anxiety.

It is also important to keep a diary. Write down things as they happen, because major events can reoccur and they have patterns that you can identify if you have the previous occurrence written down.

I included one in my own funny file.

Learn how to doodle. Have a multicolored pen handy, and if you are in class or at a conference or such, just start doodling. Draw pictures that help you remember and understand what your teacher is saying, pictures that have meaning for you. A picture is worth a thousand words and those thousand words will help you not only remember what you were thinking about, but even what you were thinking subconsciously at the time.

Then there is what the Bible recommends, and that is to be more like a child. Learn to play, to enjoy yourself and life. When you go to work, don't go to "work," for work can be depressing, but go to "play." You will get through life (and work) much easier that way.

4. Record Your Dreams

Put a pen beside your bed and record the dreams you have at night. It is while you sleep that your subconscious talks to you, when everything else has quieted down. You are more into the right side of your brain at this point, with your inhibitions down. You can say something to someone in your life here that you never would in life, things that have been building up inside you that you of which you were never even consciously aware. Your brain is trying to solve the problems you could not solve during the day.

Every time you wake up from a dream, quickly jot down a few notes about what you have dreamt. During the day you can look back into your dream diary for any patterns you recognize. You might even discover the solution to something that has been eluding you.

Once upon a time, a lady come in to our office and I told her to record what her dreams were about because she did not see the relevance of what was actually happening in them. I told her what I felt was going on before I looked at what her diary said, and sure enough it was exactly what I had told her; that she didn't appreciate herself and could never satisfy herself even while other people were satisfied with her. Her dreams had to do with being in an office; she and her husband were all disheveled, papers were all over the place, rugs and carpets were all wrong. In fact, nothing in the dream was in its proper place. She had no problem with her husband arranging one side of the office. She said *"Oh, you did such a wonderful job. How did you do that?"* She felt that she could not please anybody! She could do the best that she possibly could and still not please herself, even while everybody else is quite pleased with her in the first place.

This type of person has a tendency to become very angry at herself and see herself as extremely devalued in life, because in her mind she never meets up to the expectations of other people. However, this often indicates someone who is actually dealing with selfish issues, who needs to gain a fresh perspective from the point of view of the significant others in her life. We tend to look at ourselves through distorted mirrors, but it is very helpful and healthy to listen to the positive encouragement from other people who care about us.

Consider the great minds of scientists and inventors such as Einstein, Edison, and Da Vinci. These men knew how to originate ideas through their dreams that were amazing. Always write down your ideas and dreams. You may be amazed too.

You can also get rid of pain by doing mind exercises because pain is a perception; it is your mind's perception of what's actually going on, so if you can get rid of your perception and look at it from another perspective, then you can decrease your pain. I like using colored pens because it is very important to involve color, and the mind responds to shape, color, humor, and to size. For instance, I will tell people to color red, if it is really extreme pain. For less pain, it is orange, then yellow, blue, and finally green is my peaceful color. I put it on a scale, with green being a zero, red is a 10, and the rest fall somewhere in between.

I will also tell them to look at their pain and put it in a box. Is that box the size of this county? Is that box the size of the state? Is that box the size of this nation? Is that box the size of the world, the universe and so on. It just gives them a measure of being able to control their issue, whatever their issue is, and just to recognize that it is all energy. When the energy and the need to have that energy dissipates, so does the pain.

5. Get Your Problem Solving Team

The fifth thing is to develop a problem solving team. You get an imaginary group of people together; they can be dead, they can be alive, they can even be cartoon characters. Get these people and meet with them each morning after you get up, then sit down with them and plan the day.

If you are faithful and show up every day, they usually show up with you. Then you just present your opinions for the day and what you think is going on and allow them to make funny comments for example. It allows you to take the perception off yourself and look at it from another person's perspective, which allows for a tremendous shifting to take place. It also activates the right side of the brain that again allows your body to heal. The funnier it is, the more outrageous it is, the better. Just make sure you are not doing this exercise in front of someone, looking like a fool; that could be a big problem!

6. The Room Experiment

I do this one often. Go to your favorite room, wherever you would normally sit, and then close your eyes and imagine what is in that room. You would be shocked to know that you sometimes do not even know what color the carpet is on your floor, or the wallpaper color. You may not know where things are like special pictures, because we seldom observe what we see every day. We need to become like children and learn how to observe. Children are very observant of you, watching every move you make, everything you say, recording everything. They are also at a maximum capacity for creativity and imagination, with an unlimited belief system and nearly endless energy. Become like them and be more observant. The room experiment can be a very powerful thing.

7. Dream Board

The seventh exercise called a dream map or dream board is very important. My wife and I did this about 12 years ago and nearly 90% of the things that we put on the board have happened, including this book. Put up a board where you can post things; things you want or desire, places you want to go, experiences you want to have, goals you want to achieve. You must have a purpose, a mission in life, because this allows the attraction to take place that attracts it into your life in the first place. When you have that mission and purpose set, write them down and post them on the board. Place pictures or drawings that give vision to the dream. It does not have to make sense; it is your desires for your life, whatever they may be. Your dream board will then be there for you to look at every day, a visual reminder of what you are striving to obtain. This exercise gets the heart involved in your goals. If you just put yourself in the heart of your desires , miracles can occur. The mind can be struggling for a goal, but it will not do any good unless the heart is involved.

A dream board can have colors in it, anything that stimulates the connection of the unknown future with the goals that you have in your life. Whatever works, it does not really matter. It is yours and only yours, and it is something you can keep up for years and come back to repeatedly. The dream board correlation will shock you in how your life actually unfolds.

The Physical Exercises

Remember that I said the best time to exercise is early in the morning, when your Cortisol level is high. You need to improve your oxygen flow and clear the mind.

Swimming

One of the most powerful exercises is swimming, because it involves the entire body. It is a wonderful exercise that can really help you, but swim with caution, because pools are usually chlorinated, and one absorbs more chlorine by bathing or swimming than drinking water. The real problem is with the chlorine disinfectant byproduct. Have you ever been at a pool relaxing on a nice summer day and noticed the haze above the pool? This innocent haze is not good. This is chloroform gas you are breathing, a trihalomethane. Not only does the skin absorb the chlorine upon contact, chloroform can also cause dizziness, respiratory distress, headache, and nervous system problems. Chronic exposure can even lead to liver and kidney damage. Most of the available bio products you can use are actually organic residues that chlorine reacts too, which is more dangerous than the chlorine itself. A chlorine alternative product I sometimes recommend is Baquacil, which works by a peroxide mechanism. There are also ionic agents as well as salt-water pools, which are much safer than chlorine.

The Rebounder

If you are not a swimmer or if you have not built that in ground pool in the backyard yet, you might consider the Rebounder. It is available in most sporting goods stores and it is relatively inexpensive. The Rebounder is a mini trampoline that sits up about 9 inches off the floor, 3 or 4 feet wide. Using it will increase circulation, move accumulated toxic garbage from your cells out through your lymphatic system, and filter toxins and intruders out of your body. Using the Rebounder is not a whole lot of work, and that is why I like it. You just bounce up and down with your arms at your sides; up against gravity, holding for a brief moment in a zero-gravity point, then back down again.

Rebounding increases the gravitational forces against your body, propels many energetic vibrations through it, and not only activates the lymphatic system for its daily garbage cleaning, but exercises your organs as well. It increases breathing capacity and oxygenation, helps with cardiovascular problems due to inflammation, improves blood pressure, lowers cholesterol, and reduces insulin resistance. It also improves neuromuscular coordination in the body, increases digestion, and is great for fighting depression. If you really want to do yourself some good and minimize injury caused by bouncing wrong on your feet, I recommend the Cellcerciser brand.

Tai Chi and Yoga

There are other good exercises, of course. Anything that improves circulation is good, anything involving movement. You could get involved in the martial arts or tai chi with its fluid movements and controlled breathing. Yoga is also good, not only for stretching, but you can release extra weight as well.

People often come to the clinic to lose weight and I often ask them if they want to lose weight? They usually say "Yeah." Then I tell them there are two things in life I do not like: losing weight and growing old. When was the last time you lost something and were happy about it? It is usually painful, as is growing old, so I do not believe in either one.   I prefer to "release" the extra weight.

Walking

I recommend walking, but not jogging. Jogging is too traumatic on the joints and hips, particularly for women, and you want to avoid that in any sort of exercise. Walking, or biking, are both easy on the joints. Of course, you must do something that you enjoy, and the key is to have good ventilation. Walking or biking around outside is a good way to get all of this, taking in the neighborhood as you pass on by.

Low Resistance Training

Low resistance training is also important, something to build the muscles and get rid of excess fat. Keep it light, 4 to 6 pounds, less if that is what you are comfortable with; just do not get too comfortable, but do not get too aggressive with it either. Do it three minutes at a time. You should also alternate, a light workout one day then a heavy workout the next.

Whichever exercise you do, having a mental presence is important. You can release more weight and more effectively improve your body. Picture in your mind the workout you are giving your body, how it will shape you up. When you involve your mind and your creativity, your exercises will become much easier. People think wrongly that everything has to be difficult, that exercise cannot be fun. That is just simply wrong. You can make it fun, and when you do, it goes from being a chore to more of a habit that becomes an integral part of your daily routine.

The Case Of Kellie Bosarge

My name is Kellie. I was looking for a natural health practitioner to help with my condition, and found Dr. Lucky through a friend. I came to him with thyroid problems; I was having migraines 3 to 4 times a week, extreme fatigue, and a swollen thyroid. I was only 35 at the time.

As is usual for Dr. Lucky, he refused to let me tell him the problem. Instead, he read my body, looking for signs of what was out of balance. He was able to tell me exactly what I had been going through just from looking me over.

His solution was to put me on a nutritional program, tell me what to eat and what not to eat. Gluten was a no-no. He also gave me vitamins and other supplements; a total of 4 I had to take on a daily basis. It was not long before I showed improvement and the nearly complete disappearance of my swollen thyroid.

That was 5 years ago. Two months ago, after a year and a half of not seeing him, my thyroid was extremely swollen; a repeat of my past problems. He then went into my genetic background, and was able to pinpoint where something traumatic from my past happened. I was shocked, because it was indeed of a time when a certain event had a highly emotional effect on me.

He then performed what he called "spiritual surgery". He would pray over me, pantomiming doing actual surgery. Maybe it was because he got me to believe in him so much, or maybe something else, but my thyroid deflated back down to normal and is still down.

I also took my son to see him. Dr. Lucky pinpointed his asthma and other problems without being told. He also found some emotional issues. My son had just started preschool and was suffering from separation anxiety. Dr. Lucky gave my son a prayer to say everyday for a week to fix him up. Now my son loves school and no longer suffers from anxiety.

The Doctor's Notes:

Thirty-five years young, white female, Kellie's case involved a 2.5 inch by 2.5 inch goiter that stuck out ¾ inch from neck, which had been present about seven years. Life stressed her and her family out. I first saw her 07/2008 and evaluated her bio-energetically and found that she had a weak thyroid, sleep issues, and a problem with the right ovary. An exam revealed the thyroid goiter. We worked on a belief that was not hers but due to the constellation of ancestors in her family, and performed Present Therapy technique. Instantly the goiter decreased by about 90% while in the office and left minimal right side prominence really only seen with the hyperextension of neck. By 06/01/2011, she was doing great and had stated that the swelling was still gone but she had not paid attention to it. She then went and looked in the mirror and could see no swelling. Thank God!

This case indicates the spontaneity of the body when it is ready to heal.

The invention of doing emotional surgery began with two patients. The first was a nice gentleman who had been on oxygen for 20 years and came to me for help while he was taking several medications. He was extremely skeptical of what I was doing and became more skeptical when I told him I would be doing surgery on his bladder. I proceeded to aggravate him by telling him I had no idea how much it will cost and have never performed surgery in my life except for closing a wound. He thought I was crazy, but then I explained the connection between the lungs and the bladder and we were in the time of the bladder cycle. I told him I would do it in the chair and there would be no blood loss because I would only be holding his hand. We used a virtual cystoscope and when I told him he had an enlarged prostate and I had to remove this he perked up to a deep breath and stated he had not breathed this way in twenty years. When we started, his O2 saturation was 89% on 2L and when he left it was 96% on RA. Of course, he left his Oxygen tank with me and went home.

The second patient was a young lady whom I was asked to see by a friend. I had no knowledge of what she was dealing with, but from the way she was leaning, I thought she had severe hemorrhoids. I proceeded to find out what was wrong and the body showed a thyroid issue, bladder issue, and musculoskeletal issue, but no colon or hemorrhoid issues. I performed emotional surgery on her by working on the thyroid, balloon in bladder, and under virtual spinal anesthesia, we went to L4 and placed virtual cement in the disk place. We also prayed over her and my wife asked her to stand up and she did so with full range of motion. She was less surprised than I was because our 4-hour visit was essentially over in 15 minutes. She then told me her story.

She had been in horrible pain for over 2 years. She was driving down the highway when she felt paralyzed and had bladder difficulties. She was rushed to the hospital and diagnosed with a condition called cauda equina syndrome and had emergency surgery to remove a disk, but due to a problem with her insurance they did not replace the disk.

Emotional surgery put them in the present state with right brain dominant. The contrast of these two cases is striking. In the first case, the man was very skeptical, while in the second case I was more skeptical than the lady.

The Case Of Ruth Inmans,
As told by Majory McElroy

Ruth is 92 years old, with two types of cancer. The traditional doctors said she had cancer but she did not believe them. When she finally went to Dr. Lucky, she was ready to die.

She smoked, drank, was weak, had no strength, and always sat in the wheelchair never trying to get up. She lived alone and had people like me to come in and make her meals, bathe her, that sort of thing. On a scale of 1 to 10, with 10 being really bad, she was an 8, both physically and emotionally. Dr. Lucky took one look at her and picked up on all of this.

Dr. Lucky changed her diet, putting her on whole foods and nutritional products. He also addressed her emotional issues, worked with her to give her some positive feedback and how she could help herself. Her son had just passed away and her daughter was sick, and that put her into a depressed mood. Dr. Lucky worked to give her a more positive attitude to help her improve.

On her first follow-up visit she was on very few medications. He gave her regular treatments with light that helped her get up and down and get rid of parasites.

After three weeks she got up, took her own shower, and got stronger. Now, on a scale of 1 to 10, she rates herself at a 2 to 4. She is concerned about extending her life now and is a lot happier.

Dr. Lucky treats the whole body. He does not diagnose for a disease but sees what the whole body is lacking and fixes that first; that in turn fixes the other symptoms. He uses both his left and right brain in treatment and diagnosis, talks in layman terms, and is a good listener that sees the overall picture immediately. He gives patients his undivided attention, and is truly interested in a patient's health, calling his patients to check up on them. A caring compassionate person who gives away more than he takes in, he is an unusual phenomenon.

The Doctor's Notes:

Ruth is a 92 years young, white female with a history of leukemia, years of heavy smoking, and is very matter-of-fact. She is hard of hearing secondarily to her young age, and treated recently for hyperthyroidism with radioactive iodine ablation and synthroid replacement. She stated that she felt terrible and was very agitated by the amount of pain that had kept her in the bed or in the recliner all the time, except to use the bedside potty. The pain was in the lower back without radiation. She was not able to have an x-ray secondarily to the severe pain. She told me she did not trust doctors and came to me to prepare to die so she could meet Jesus. She rated her pain "20 on a scale of 1 to10 sonny." Emotionally, she was concerned about her grandchild and his future without her. She does not like the political situation this country is in, and what they are going to do to the elderly.

I then told her the cigarette smoke was about to take my breath away and I usually invest hours to evaluate patients, but I am afraid I would be dead by then. So we got right to the point: *"What can I do?"* Again, she stated that she wanted to be able to be out of pain and use her own toilet and then she could meet Jesus. She did not want to change any habits. I explained to her that she did not only have leukemia, but bone involvement as well as colon malignancy. She stated she knew, but she just wanted to meet the Lord. She did not want any pain medicine and that is why she came to see me; to die without pain.

In March of 2009, the patient was extremely cachectic, wasting severe kyphosis, pale complexion, and obviously chronically sick. She was hard of hearing and talked very loud with very little tact. I told her I would do a quick bioenergetic exam and imprint the nutritional agents with phototherapy. Amazingly, after the session, her hands she could not previously move from her lap could now be raised. I asked her to focus on the goal of getting to the "potty" by herself.

Two weeks later, she got up, went to the blinds, and tried to open them. She continued the imprint and phototherapy and was able to use her toilet.

She returned to my office for a visit in June of 2009 and was happy that she did not have much pain at all, but her appetite was lacking. She stated that she had two different kinds of cancer and still wanted to meet Jesus. She was still smoking at that time.

Her exam was very kyphotic, and her complexion had improved some and she was now able to stand. According to her helper, she did not use the wheelchair much except for transportation. We continued phototherapy, Laser Energy Detoxification (LED), and visualization. She wanted to be able to shower herself.

She came again in September of 2009, and continued to do much better and took a shower for the first time since March 2009. Her color and disposition were greatly improved. Her nutritional supplement needs have decreased since we have been imprinting. Her only complaint was not being able to distinguish words clearly when a person speaks to her. We used LED, Zinc, B vitamins, and Omega 3 in April of 2010; She stated her fingernails which have always been thin as paper had become hard and she had stopped smoking in February so she "could get to heaven." Patient had been fairly well and concerned about prolonging her life. Now, she still wants to meet Jesus, but knows she will not die until she finishes her purpose.

The moral of the story: Do not go to a prolongevity doctor if you want to die!

" The doctor of the future will no longer treat the human frame with drugs, but rather will cure and prevent disease with nutrition. "

-Thomas Edison

Chapter FOUR

7 Supplements To Extend Your Life

he key to longevity is to reduce inflammation. Inflammation is part of everything related to the process of aging, and aging is the only disease that I choose to acknowledge because it should not be going on in the first place. Heart disease or malignancy causes the majority of death in our country. Which are 95% avoidable if you take the right preventive measures. With the right supplements in your diet, you can reduce inflammation and improve your longevity.

For this purpose, I have come up with the seven of the most important nutritional supplements that you should have in your diet. All of them are very inexpensive and quite easy to get. Some of them may already be in your diet, although the way food is over-processed, treated with pesticides, hormones, and what not, that may not always be true, regardless of what the label says. Even if you eat a good diet and take a good multivitamin, you should include the following supplements.

1. Glyconutrients

The number one supplement that will help extend your life is glyconutrients. These are sugars attached to either proteins or lipids in the body. They provide for the communication between cells. When cells communicate, it is as if they shake hands with one another. These proteins are the hands they shake with, allowing for the cell signaling mechanism to occur. As such, they play a key role in every metabolic process that involves cellular communication, which is about every metabolic process. In pregnancy, for instance, when the sperm and the egg come together in a 500,000-volt blast, that energetic process is mediated by glyco proteins. From birth to death, glyco proteins are there.

When cells encounter one another, they read the proteins on one another's cell membranes, which consist of certain sugars. If the cell detects the wrong sugars on the neighboring cell, it is assumed to be a foreign invader. We obtain plenty of sugar in our diet, too much in fact, but most of it are the wrong **types** of sugars. We obtain far too much Glucose, for example. The body attacks cells that are missing the right sugars as foreign invaders. Thus, we get the autoimmune diseases from rheumatory arthritis to fibromyalgia.

Your body is able to make the proper sugars, but the mechanism by which it does so is extremely energy intensive, so if you do not have enough energy then you become deficient in these sugars. Glyconutrients do what all these other sugars do, maintain a proper balance of the right sugars, keep your energy up, and make sure that cells can properly recognize one another. Glyconutrients are immune modulators, increasing the immune system when underactive and depressing the immune system when overactive. This benefit makes them very important.

My first encounter with glyconutrients was when I was living in Washington State and my brother called me from 3000 miles away. My father had a systolic blood pressure in the 70s, severe chills, and was incoherent. My family prayed over him and I called in for antibiotics for the acute pyelonephritis and told them to double the dose. He did not go to the hospital and God healed him with recovery of his health.

Later, I witnessed another attack because he was having them about once a month. This time I placed him on D-mannose, which I had heard about from Dr. Jonathan Wright. He took small amounts routinely, and over the past 12 years has only had two urinary tract infections, and that is when he stops taking the D-mannose or runs out and does not tell anyone. For an E-coli infection, D-mannose competes with the bacteria for the receptor on the bladder wall, and drinking water with it will eliminate the bacteria. Cranberry's active ingredient is also D-mannose but less of it. D-mannose has several other functions helpful for the body as well.

One has to be careful while taking these powerful nutrients and keep a close eye on blood pressure and blood sugar, especially if you are on medication because they can drop fast. I have patients that start and their blood sugar begins to climb during their morning fasting; they say that their blood sugar is "getting worse on this stuff." I tell them, *"Hallelujah, your blood sugar is falling too low due to your medicine while you sleep and we need to decrease the amount of medicine you are taking in the evening."* They seem pretty happy with the idea, and the morning blood sugar falls as a result.

Other times people using glyconutrients may see an initial increase in their sugar level because the glyconutrients are actually clearing off the walls of the blood vessels, but if they continue taking the supplement, they will notice their sugar actually starting to decline. That is an important thing to note when you are on glyconutrients.You can get glyconutrients in mushrooms, the aloe plant, seaweed, or you can get it in a more convenient supplement form that costs about $8.00 a month.

2. Garlic

Garlic is the next life extending supplement, and a tasty one it is, though if you want to avoid the burning, eat a banana with it. Eat part of one clove, then a piece of a banana, followed by another piece of the clove, until it is all gone.

Known as Russian penicillin, it is antibiotic, antiviral, anti-parasitic, and antifungal. It also helps improve blood sugar by reducing insulin resistance, which is heavily associated with aging. Garlic also protects cell membranes from free radical damage, working together with glyconutrients in this respect. Garlic helps also in the membranes lining the blood vessels, preventing everything from excess calcium to cholesterol from building up and causing blood and heart problems. Garlic prevents the chain of events that lead to the maladies of arterial buildup and bad cholesterol. In fact, it also prevents the oxidation of cholesterol from happening in the first place.

Garlic keeps tissues elastic, improves blood flow, and prevents cardiac issues. If you are interested in the complexities of these cardiac issues, then read on; otherwise, just go to the next topic.

Garlic's key component is something called *S-allylcysteine*, which is a sulphur moiety. This has great importance as it inhibits malignancy and promotes cardiovascular health by providing for significant protection against oxidation of the membranes. Peroxidase enzymes that actually cause free radical damage and destruction of the membranes attack the cell membranes. Garlic and the glyconutrients magnify the benefit, because this is the location where the glycoprotein and lipids are present... outside the cell membrane. They also work at the endothelial level where there is a thin layer of cells. Endothelial cell dysfunction is one of the common causes of heart attacks, which allows for the calcium and all the bad stuff to get in through the cell membrane to the inner part of the intimae and start causing problems.

The intimae are composed of three layers: the endothelial, the interstitial, and the elastic component. This is where so many problems originate – from the initial fracture of plaque in coronary artery disease. The process of coronary artery occlusion occurs when there is plaque build up from the calcium, the fibrin, and the platelets; all of this turns into a big mess, then macrophages and white blood cells take up all this debris and die and become something called foam cells. They even change the smooth muscle part of the blood vessel as well.

When you can actually stop it from getting in there in the first place, then you have made a huge difference and helped to prevent atherosclerosis, which leads to cardiovascular disease. The problem is not necessarily cholesterol, but rather oxidized LDL cholesterol. We will look at this in more detail when we talk about Vitamin C and how it works in this mechanism.

Garlic function protects the cell membrane, but it also reduces the blood coagulatability. This is another great benefit because when you have heart disease, you have toxic blood, which means the blood flow slows down, becomes thickened, and you have reduced clotting ability.

Garlic helps increase the blood flow that increases oxygen to the cells, thus preventing oxidative stress and reducing free radicals at the cell level. When you talk vascular health, you talk garlic.

Garlic also prevents the oxidation of the cholesterol from occurring in the first place, so LDL cholesterol is actually great. Cholesterol is just an innocent bystander. It is not something that is really aggressive and problematic. It simply indicates there is a problem going on and it needs attention and repair. When there is a problem, the body signals the liver to start producing cholesterol to ward that off from happening. Garlic reduces the mediators that bring in more platelets that lead to thickening and cause the heart attack to happen in the first place.

Garlic also increases nitric oxide. Nitric oxide is important in the dilatation of tissue, which is a very important factor because if your vessels do not vasodilate, and you have heart and artery problems in addition to the lack of elasticity, then you do not get the oxygen you need. Garlic improves blood flow and thus oxygenation.

You can take garlic every day. It does not hurt anybody. There are no risks associated with it. However, as with any nutrient, use caution and consult your doctor if using other medications that have similar effects on the blood vessels. If you are taking a blood thinning medication, which is common, the garlic could lead to increased thinning, which could cause issues.

All the nutrients suggested here require someone that has some knowledge of how medicines interact with nutrients. With other supplements, anything that thins the blood, there is this possibility. In my personal experience, Ginkgo Biloba, Ginseng, and even Ginger can cause issues with thinning of blood, but the most common medications to be aware of are Warfarin, Coumadin, and Plavix.

Garlic should be a part of everybody's diet. It is just absolutely fantastic…except for the smell, and for that, you can get a tongue brush from the store to scrape the smell away. Bad breath is a small price to pay for the good it does. It is much more beneficial to take it than not.

3. Magnesium

Magnesium is one of the six elements in the periodic table that is essential for your body to function properly, yet nearly everyone is deficient in it. If we rely on the lab, we may get skewed results because 99% of Magnesium is in the bone, 1% in the blood. So, when the lab measures your magnesium levels, they are only measuring the amount in the blood. The bones hold on to Magnesium until the situation becomes dire; I call it the "Rob Peter to pay Paul" phenomenon. Stress depletes magnesium as well as nearly every medication (diuretics, steroid hormones, beta-blockers, proton pump inhibitors [the purple pill] and many more). Just the simple things in life that increase cortisol, such as stress, will deplete Magnesium. If you drink caffeinated beverages, they are depleting your Magnesium. We are seeing an epidemic proportion of magnesium deficiency. Worse yet, since magnesium is not usually in our diets, it is very difficult to replenish.

Magnesium is involved in close to 300 different functions in the body, and it interacts with over 300 different enzymes. It is fundamental in helping your body produce ATP, which is the energy reserve of your cells and your metabolism; it gives you the power and energy that you need actually to have life. Here are a few examples:

- Magnesium protects from coronary artery disease, by shielding the arterial linings from sudden stress.
- Magnesium is also important for healthy muscles because calcium and magnesium operate actin and myosin involved in muscle contraction.
- Low magnesium or calcium can cause cramping in the legs and a heart attack affecting a large muscle called the heart.
- When someone is under stress, it opens up calcium channels, which allows calcium to influx and cause a process called Saponification. This is not good. This has a negative effect on the Lipid panel, which influences cholesterol.
- Magnesium is important for supporting the non-oxidized LDL, preventing it from oxidizing and fulfilling its role as the "bad" cholesterol.

- Magnesium is important for glucose tolerance factor, along with chromium and B vitamins, which help in insulin resistance by reducing inflammation and promoting longevity.
- Magnesium is the drug of choice for Torsades De Pointes, a life-threatening emergency during which doctors administer it via an IV push.
- Magnesium is helpful for calming the nervous system, avoiding respiratory diseases, headaches, and eclampsia.

Many foods contain magnesium such as green vegetables, nuts, and seafood. However, the stress and the junk food in our lives almost completely deplete any magnesium that is in our body. Furthermore, too often we do not take supplements until it is too late because our Magnesium level does not reflect the deficiency. The ideal level is between 2-4 mg/dl. Cardiac instability can occur when a person's magnesium level is less than 2 mg/dl. At this level, the heart draws on the bone reserves, promoting osteoporosis related to heart disease. Therefore, one of the best ways to measure heart disease is to measure bone density to find out what is really going on at the bone level and if they are losing these wonderful cofactors that support bone as well as heart health. Bottom line: It is a very essential element and a wonderful supplement.

Magnesium supplements come in a number of different forms. I do not recommend Magnesium Oxide, because Magnesium Oxide is very poorly absorbed; out of 400 mg you may get 20 mg absorbed, so it's really not doing you much good when you need, for example, 180 milligrams. Magnesium IV is another form that assists in situations where it is critical to settle a person down, like if they have heart issues, ischemic, someone with Delirium Tremens; any situation where you need to settle down the nervous system.

Magnesium has a very low toxicity; you could give someone 16 grams of it and most people will still be deficient. All the problematic conditions associated with low magnesium will resolve with replacement, but it can take time.

I have a story about the importance of Magnesium in my residency that led me to think holistically. Only God and magnesium saved this man's life. He was supposed to die the next day and was DNR (do not resuscitate) and I was on the code team, so I always made the nurses' lives absolutely "Heaven." When I was on duty, they did not want to deal with me, but they had to call me because I was captain of the code team that night. They said, *"This man is dying,"* and I would go up there and say, *"Well, what can I do for him? He's dying." "Very good, we know." "Well let me look at his chart."* I looked at his chart, and then called in some kind of wild order like Magnesium to someone in kidney failure. He's on a ventilator, 100% oxygen, O$_2$ saturation in the 60's, his heart rate is 200, and he's in liver failure, kidney failure, and there's no apparent hope for him. The nurses phoned my residency assistant dean at 2:00 am, woke him up and said, *"This guy's trying to kill a patient,"* then they call the CEO of the hospital. Finally, I got the okay and by morning, we had him weaned off the ventilator, his liver functions were normal and the kidney functions improved by half. He went home 3 days later. I said, *"Well I guess you got stopped from going celestially home by just one simple agent, Magnesium."*

4. Vitamin D and Vitamin K

A couple of vitamins that are essential in longevity are Vitamin D and Vitamin K. Cholesterol conversion occurs to Vitamin D by sun exposure, but there are people who get plenty of sunlight exposure who do not get enough Vitamin D. Sunscreen blocks the conversion process but even my clients who do not use sunscreen have Vitamin D deficiency. Perhaps something is going on with the atmosphere that is preventing UVB (ultraviolet) light radiation needed to convert cholesterol into Vitamin D.

Another problem is that too many people are on medications, such as cholesterol drugs, that interfere with cholesterol levels, which are important for all the lipid soluble hormones in the body. By taking these medications, they can become deficient in almost all of their hormones, increasing the risk of malignancies.

If you do get adequate levels of sunlight, Vitamin D research shows a reduction in the incidence of prostate, ovarian, colon, and breast malignancies. The research also indicates an improvement in immune conditions of all kinds and is an anti-tuberculosis agent. It is also important for bones, heart health, and is a natural ace inhibitor.

One client came to our office who had a Vitamin D level of less than five. She was African American, which contributed to the problem because she did not completely absorb vitamin D due to the increased melanin in her skin that was hindering the absorption of Vitamin D. She had a blood pressure reading of about 200 over 110. She was on blood pressure medicine. We simply gave her 50,000 units of Vitamin D (which I do not recommend unless you are under the watchful eye of a physician) and when she returned home, her blood pressure had dropped to 120 over 70 for the first time in years. The moral of the story: Vitamin D is a very effective blood pressure reducing agent!

There are some risks. People with Sarcoidosis, which is an immune problem, may need to avoid taking Vitamin D. They may have *lymphoproliferative* conditions such as lymphoma, and taking Vitamin D could make this worse.

Most people do not have issues with Vitamin D supplementation. It is a fat-soluble vitamin, so there is a degree of toxicity, but usually it takes a huge amount of Vitamin D to get toxic. 2000 units of Vitamin D should be fine for most people. I use Lab Corp to measure Vitamin D level. The ideal hydroxyvitamin D level is 50-60 ng/ml

After getting the initial lab work, take vitamin D3, then obtain the second level 2 to 3 months later, particularly in the winter when people become very deficient of sunlight and almost all of us require Vitamin D to get through flu season.

Then there is Vitamin K. Vitamin K is actually Vitamin K2. There are three types of Vitamin K: Vitamin K1, Vitamin K2, and Vitamin K3. Vitamin K2 is menaquinone and fermented soybean product called Natto contain Vitamin K2. Intestinal bacteria produce Vitamin K2 so we have to be careful when doctors prescribe anti-biotics.

We surely know that Vitamin K is part of the blood clotting mechanics, but it also helps in several other areas:

- It helps control calcium absorption. Vitamin K grabs calcium, directs it to the bones and prevents it from building up in the blood vessels. This is good for preventing osteoporosis.
- It helps prevent kidney stones from forming (caused by calcium leaching out of the bones).
- It is doubly helpful in people over 50, because that is when the acidity of the stomach starts decreasing making the absorption of nutrients more difficult. The body attempts to replenish this deficiency by pulling calcium out of the bones and putting it where the body needs it most.
- Vitamin K acts as an anti-inflammatory agent. It inhibits the IL 6 production and this is really important in aging because it is inflammation in general that causes the aging process.
- Osteocalcin is one of the bone markers that indicates how your bones are working. Vitamin K2 activates osteocalcin so it will absorb the calcium into the bone in the first place.
- Vitamin K is best known as a clotting agent, but before you start thinking that too much Vitamin K will lead to too much clotting, the body simply flushes out any it does not need, so no need to worry.

People on blood thinners are depleting themselves of Vitamin K, leading to bone fragility and increasing the risk of bone and hip fractures. Vitamin K will harden the bones and soften the arteries, but Vitamin D will harden the bones and also the arteries...if you take too much.

You need about 45 milligrams of Vitamin K, which is a substantial amount, but there is no risk in taking this amount. It is a hormone type vitamin, as is Vitamin D, and both are very inexpensive. For people that are on Coumadin or other blood thinners, I highly recommend that you contact your physician before even using Vitamin K.

5. Vitamin C

The next life extending supplement is Vitamin C. It has a tremendous impact on the immune system and is one of the most powerful antioxidants around.

We know that Scurvy results from a Vitamin C deficiency. James Lind discovered Vitamin C and its relationship with Scurvy. He would take his subjects to the edge of death and then just give them some lemon rinds and they would become healthy again. He concluded that the power of Vitamin C increased the immune system to tremendous levels.

The mechanism by which this happens is that it increases the Glutathione Level, which is one of the most powerful antioxidants under the sun. We cannot take some Glutathione orally secondarily to the stomach acid breaking it down. However, when you take enough Vitamin C, the Glutathione levels increase preventing lipid peroxidation activity, which is a culprit in cell membrane breakdown. Vitamin C is a very powerful antioxidant that increases glutathione, and is necessary for Vitamin E to be absorbed, which helps to reduce oxidative stress.

Vitamin C is also good for collagen and the cardiovascular system. Collagen contains Glycine, Lysine, Proline, Hydroxyproline and Arginine; there must be cross-linkage in order to have healthy collagen. Otherwise, if you do not have enough Vitamin C, a cross linkage deficiency will occur that allows amino acid to be exposed, which causes the body to attack itself. Sometimes, coronary artery disease is simply the body attacking itself, just like inflammation. When the body searches for immune cells to counter-attack, there is a compound that can be measured (like lipoprotein A) that begins to increase. This reaction causes all the inflammatory cells to rush in and cause oxidized LDL. But the Vitamin C protects the oxidation of LDL and allows for the Proline and Lysine amino acids not to be exposed, which in turn inhibits the formation of the collagen, which would have otherwise initiated the cardiovascular condition. You can see the power of this Vitamin C.

It also helps with any type of malignancy. In general, a malignant cell has 25 times more glucose receptors on it than a normal cell. Glucose looks much like Vitamin C. When the malignant cells see the Vitamin C, they think it is glucose so they take the Vitamin C instead of the glucose. Then, as a potent antioxidant, the Vitamin C goes into the malignant cells and neutralizes the toxins or free radicals in the body that are causing the problems in the first place. Your cells then create the acidity needed for the malignant cell to kill itself, but it does not affect normal cells in this way. Vitamin C protect the normal cells, so it has an oxidative stress that's good for the body which means it's a pro-oxidant as well as an antioxidant, which is another powerful part to the Vitamin C paradigm.

Vitamin C also helps lower cholesterol. Many people need more Vitamin C, as well as B Vitamins to help support their healthy cholesterol. You will see their cholesterol come down as well as triglycerides and fasting insulin. It is also important for improving blood sugars.

Too much Vitamin C can lead to problems, such as kidney stones due mainly to all the citric components, but this is very rare. Vitamin C deficiency sometimes causes kidney stones not vice versa. There is often a double edged sword to anything that you take into your body, but the benefits of this supplement far far outweigh the risk, even if you take 1000 milligrams a day.

You absorb about 200 milligrams of Vitamin C if taken orally. Even if you consume 10,000 milligrams there should not be a problem. If you take too much, all that will happen is some diarrhea as the body flushes the excess out. I take about 1000 milligrams of crystal Vitamin C for better absorption. Take Vitamin C as calcium ascorbate, or magnesium ascorbate, but I caution you about obtaining it from corn because corn is genetically modified about 90% of the time, which is not good. Liposomal Vitamin C is another good alternative, almost equivalent to getting it from a hospital IV. You should not be afraid to take 1000 mg a couple times a day.

6. Iodine

The sixth life extending supplement is iodine. Usually taken in the form of potassium iodide, iodine works with the thyroid. You only need about 3 milligrams for the thyroid to work. Most of the iodines on the market are 5% elemental iodine, which have an impact on the breasts, ovaries, and prostate, so this can be a health concern. Lugol's Solution is 10% potassium iodide, to support and protect the thyroid, and 5% elemental iodine in 85% water, to support the breasts, ovaries, and prostate.

Iodine is a halide, as are Bromine, Chlorine, and Fluorine, so they can compete with each other, which is the danger of having all these toxic substances around. They can displace the iodine and cause significant issues with the thyroid in general. About 70% of people are iodine deficient. In the Japanese culture, though, they take about 12 milligrams of iodine a day in their diet, so the 50 micrograms recommended by the RDA is actually very deficient. There is some risk with iodine, however, so you will definitely want to talk to a physician before taking it.

Disclaimer: The latest Fukushima disaster regarding radiation release into the waters and air around the nuclear reactors in Japan have reported that you must be careful eating seaweed, fish, and fermented soy from this part of the world.

Iodine is vital to the thyroid, but it is also a good antifungal, antivirus, and antiparasitic, and stimulates the immune system, as well as helping with insulin resistance. There are different forms of iodine. The body stores excess iodine as T4, the inactive form of iodine. Some medications will actually convert iodine into this inactive form, leading to an inactive thyroid and associated problems, including weight gain. A word of caution: Avoid artificial sweeteners, like Splenda, because they contain chlorine that competes with iodine for its place in the body.

Many doctors do not know how to read thyroid tests. They check TSH and/or T4 and that is all they follow. Many of the drugs prescribed are synthetic, in that they will increase your T4, but do very little for your T3, which is the active hormone. The TSH is affected by many things, so when I recommend doing a thyroid test. I recommend getting TSH, free T3 and free T4, instead of a TSH to determine what is going on with the thyroid, because the T3 is the active form.

Your "T" number refers to how many iodine atoms make up the hormone: T1 is one iodine atom, T2 is 2 iodine atoms, T3 is 3, and T4 is 4.

The T4 is inactive, which is the majority of the body's thyroid supply. The body makes T3 in small amounts by the thyroid and most of it from conversion of T4 in the peripheral tissues such as the liver and kidney, but the T4 stays in the inactive form. The body knows that too much iodine in the thyroid would not be a good thing, so it only allows for a very small amount of T3 to work. When someone gets too much T4, like in a situation where somebody is under excess amounts of stress, it will convert into reverse T3. They may be very sick, on several medications that interfere, by taking steroids, or on birth control. These things will convert T3 back to T4, causing the thyroid to get overloaded, resulting in an inactive thyroid. This is why some people have problems with weight gain. They have large amounts of reverse T3 stored in the liver.

Bromine sometimes substitutes for iodine, which is extremely toxic, as well as lead, chlorine, and fluorine. This is important in the Midwest where they put Bromine into milk and bread. Scientists discovered the bromine issue when people in the Midwest began developing goiters, and then later discovered it was due to a lack of iodine in the soil. The Government replaced Iodine in bread and milk and the goiter situation improved. The problem was that the government replaced the iodine in breads with bromine and other brominated products, which eliminates the iodine in the body.

I take about 3 milligrams of iodine myself, but if you have any doubts, it is best to have yourself tested to see if you have an allergy to it. Those allergic to seafood may actually be allergic to the iodine in it. A good test to see if you are allergic is to put it on your skin and see if you have a reaction. If you do not, and you have never had a bad reaction to iodine from a new type of drug, then you are probably safe to use iodine.

7. Coenzyme Q10

Coenzyme Q10 is the next significant supplement. It is important in the *mitochondria in cells, specifically in the electric transport chain to help provide energy in the form of ATP.* It is a good antioxidant used to protect the mitochondria and is a fat-soluble vitamin. Coenzyme Q10 also improves the cardiovascular output, helps the arteries, increases energy output from mitochondria, helps prevent mutations in the DNA, and suppresses inflammation.

Coenzyme Q10 deficiency increases as you age, but is also depleted by many medications, including cholesterol medicines and Statin drugs. Such heart medications will deplete Co-Q10 in the heart cells, leading to a loss of energy in the heart. The muscle cells have around 4000 to 5000 mitochondria because of the large energy requirements, which make Co-Q10 a significant player there as well.

The brain is another area where Co-Q10 can become depleted, leading to mental health issues. However, such people are probably on multiple drugs in the first place which create the Co-Q10 deficiency.

It is also an anti-malignant agent. Mitochondria have their own DNA supply, replicating itself as needed to fulfill a cell's energy requirements. It is actually bacteria in primitive form that allows for aerobic oxidation and respiration, sort of like breathing, so the cell can manifest itself. When you take Co-Q10, you are actually preventing mutations from taking place in the mitochondrial-DNA that would otherwise cause significant toxic transformation and promotion of malignancies. This initiation and promotion of the two stages of malignancy is inflammation, making Co-Q10 another longevity-promoting anti-inflammatory agent.

What depletes Co-Q10 can also deplete Magnesium, leading to leg cramps as a telltale sign, but a Co-Q10 supplement can fix this problem.

Take it with olive oil or something fat based to get the good absorption, but the best way to absorb Co-Q10 is to take it in its more active form, Ubiquinol. One study found that taking about 300 milligrams of Coenzyme Q10 for 11 days increased its level in the blood by 4 times. I recommend about 100 milligrams per day, but if you are taking blood thinning medications, then you should inform your doctor before using this supplement.

8. Bonus entry: Turmeric

This anti-inflammatory supplement is as close as your kitchen cabinet or local grocery store. Everyone should take on a daily basis. It is very safe and the only problem is that some people may be sensitive and develop nausea or diarrhea. It prevents any type of malignant transformation that might occur, and prevents metastasis (how the body spreads malignancies around). It prevents the cell signal mechanism from activating tumors, placing abnormal cells in the rest stage so the body can either kill them or undergo programmed cell death, known as apoptosis. The cell also reserves the option to repair itself and become normal.

Turmeric also has an effect on tumor necrosis factor alpha, which is a contributing factor in malignancy and inflammation. It works through the tumor suppressive gene P53, through the cell cycling.

Turmeric also helps with blood sugar control and improves heart health.

In summary turmeric is an extra one for your consideration, a popular addition to curry spice mixes. Completely safe, it prevents the spreading of malignancies around the body, reduces inflammation, helps with blood sugar, improves heart health, and is a source of Vitamins E and C. It is also quite tasty!

The Case Of Jane M.

In December of 2009, I was diabetic and had thyroid problems. My legs hurt, so I tried a chiropractor; my lower back was out of joint but the chiropractor said it was diabetes. I took the sugar test myself and did find my sugar was up. I did not sleep well because of my aching legs, and I was also overweight, at 168 pounds.

I did not want medicine so I went to Dr. Lucky, whom I'd heard of by word of mouth. At my first visit, he took about an hour and a half to examine me head to toe. He then traced my family back through my parents, and I mentioned how my daughter had a bike accident that had scarred up her face and two days later I got sick. He helped me get through that and asked my daughter to forgive herself; she now has no more scars.

He put me on a gluten-free diet, just fruits, vegetables, nuts, and lean meat. I took natural supplements, Vitamin B-12, and Vitamin D. He used a light therapy to detox me then told me to go barefoot around the house, learn to relax, and let my feet hit the grass for electrons to flow. He explained the electron flow with the use of a doll; we held hands with the doll between us to show how electrons can flow in a current through the doll.

Now my blood is down to normal, I have lost weight, and I feel a lot better. I have more energy and I workout. I am no longer considered diabetic. I send other people to him now, including my granddaughter when she got thyroid problems. She is feeling much better.

The Doctor's Notes:

Sixty-one year young, white female who saw me initially in January of 2010 with sugar issues. The doctor started her on a diet and the medical field felt she would require medicine to control blood sugar in the range of 200-300 and averaging about 220. She had eczema all over her face and conjunctival involvement, and she had been squinting her eyes for about 5 years. She used crystal light drinks that contained artificial sweeteners, and had been on high cholesterol medication for 10 years; she was on Lipitor and the doctors wanted her to change to Crestor. She was also on omeprazole for difficulty swallowing and had intermittent chest pain, took thyroid medication for low thyroid, and weighed about 168 lbs.

We put her on a gluten and dairy free diet and discontinued the artificial sweeteners and almost immediately, her blood sugars began to fall. Her left eye, which had been squinted, opened. She applied silver solution to her face, which drastically improved her eczema issue, and we placed her on bio-indentical hormones. We also discontinued the omeprazole because she was already suffering from hypochlorohydria, and placed her on compounded thyroid. We then supplemented her diet with food-based chromium, niacinamide, Vitamin D3, proteolytic enzymes, along with glyconutrients. When she returned 1 month later, her blood sugar was averaging about 120, and her weight decreased to 157 pounds. Hba1c previously 9.5 was now reduced to 6.2, 120-130 average over the past 3 months.

Other lab results:

First Visit	About 9 months later
Insulin level 19.4	14.5-still way too high
fibrinogen activity 317	267 indicates the ability to clot
Cardiac CRP 4.6	1.71 indicates risk of MI or stroke over 6mo
Vitamin D 33.8	59.5
AST 53	22
ALT 53	29
cholesterol 195 on lipitor	176 -- off cholesterol med
triglycerides 175	156
HDL 40	45 good cholesterol, so call
LDL 120	107

Even after having taken steroids by injection and by mouth for several days, along with antibiotics, she quickly recovered.

We also dealt with emotional issues of the past and did the steps to wellness outlined in this book.

The moral of the story: We must eat healthy and supplement with targeted nutritional supplements.

The Case Of Cynthia N.

I was fatigued, needed to lose weight, and did not know what to do, until I was referred to Dr. Lucky by a friend. He had me fill out a history then did a muscle test; he put something between my fingers to see if I could hold them together. He found that I was taking too many supplements, had a hormone imbalance, anemia, and thyroid problems. The blood work he ordered confirmed the diagnosis.

He put me on vitamins, iodine, and adjusted my supplements to suit my needs. He used prayer a lot, as well as the Ondamed, and dealt with some emotional issues I needed to clear up. He tries to avoid medications and heal the body overall, and goes beyond what more conventional doctors would do. I also believe that God gives him insight into one's overall health.

Before I weighed 168 pounds, now I'm at 125 and feeling a lot better and still doing what the doctor told me. He is not about the money but the love of a person, and is the kindest person you will meet.

The Doctor's Notes:

She is into pro-longevity and is a testimony of someone who was taking a laundry basket of supplements that were extremely good but excessively many. This story just emphasizes how one can release weight and not have to take a tremendous amount of supplements. Oh, and she actually did bring in a laundry basket!

" *Those who think they have no time for healthy-eating will sooner or later have to find time for illness.* "

-Edward Stanley

Chapter Five

7 Steps To Detoxifying Decades Of Pollution In Your Body

———◦◦◄◄►◄◦◦———

So many people try to lose weight and get healthy…only to fail. What they do not realize is that they have toxins in their body that they need to get rid of in order to reset their metabolism. They need to detoxify themselves. Detoxification just means a housecleaning of the body from the years of neglect and abuse that happen, a spring-cleaning of one's self. I like to do more of a superficial, gentle type cleansing than these radical cleanings that people so often get involved with; like the difference between cleaning a house with a broom versus a firehose. We gently clean the mind, the body, and the spirit all at one time.

The body is like a house, with its own electrical system, plumbing, sewer system, and the like. To get the house of your body running smoothly, you need to make sure that all of its essential components are nice and clean. The pipes must be free, wiring intact, sewage cleaned out, and so on. The purpose of this chapter is to show you how you can do some internal spring-cleaning to set your house in order.

1. Spiritual Detoxification

We start with the most important part of your house. Your spirit is the electrical system that runs the house, its power; if your electrical system is not working properly then nothing in your house is going to work either. Our beliefs can clog up our ability to process things the way we should thus hindering us from healing. You need to clean the mental garbage out, like rewiring your house or replacing the fuses, and we have several techniques to do so, some of which I have developed on my own. Spiritual issues are not something for which you can really plan; they just happen. What you have to do is reframe beliefs that are not serving you, and then you can start to heal. To begin with, you have to realize that there are different levels to the spirit, and each of these has its own needs and treatments.

The Mental Body is the first level; it is where all of our life events are recorded, our thoughts, beliefs, attitudes, and everything that we have lived through. Problems in your past, emotions you have not yet dealt with, all of this is here.

The body has about 100,000 metabolic processes going on at any one time; all of it prioritized your DNA expanding and contracting billions of times a second, all of this happening at the same frequency. Like any re-action involving vibrations, the body emits packets of energy (photons of light). This energy goes out through the cells via structures called tubu-lins that transmit the energy to the outside into a very faint field of light surrounding the person. Memories are stored in this field of light, which is important, because this is how scientists use Light Therapy to test and change the autonomic nervous system, in often immediate and dramatic ways.

In our clinic, we use variety of modalities to help with cleansing of the body, soul, and spirit. We teach meditation and visualization procedures. There are therapies for tapping into different meridians, vocal mapping, but sometimes the simplest and most important therapy is just to talk with someone. Remember that patients are people, and by talking with them, you can discover exactly what the problem is.

The Intuitive Body is the next level of the spirit; it goes beyond your own thoughts and subconscious, a collective consciousness that reaches beyond the mind; trauma, unresolved conflicts, ancestral conflicts that remained unresolved and got passed down to the next generation. This is where we look over a patient's genealogy and see what triggered their is-sue, then allow them to see that it is not their problem. We also use other therapies to clean the Intuitive Body; sound therapy, color therapy, voice mapping, and other techniques that involve a person's electromagnetic imprint and some quantum mechanics to explain, but don't worry, I won't go into those here!

The third level is the Energy Level; it is the electromagnetic field generated by the nervous system. Some people or special photography can sometimes visualize the electromagnetic field that surrounds the body; it is a person's aura. Certain electrical devices that deal with electromagnetic fields can measure and influence the electromagnetic field. Devices such as the "Ondamed", Laser Energy Detox, micro-current therapy, and other therapies that the inventors designed to improve the energy flow to the body. I will talk about these devices and therapies in a later chapter.

The last level is the level that doctors work off, which is the Physical Level. This is where more traditional doctors focus, while I deal with the other areas. Taken all together, this is how we look at the energetic system and how to improve the power running through your house.

2. Colon And Bladder Detoxification

The colon and bladder are your house's sewer system. All the garbage collected by your body goes though here, so it is essential that they remain clean. If a house's sewer backs up, you have sewage all over the place; the same goes for the colon and bladder. If a person allows the sewage from these two organs to back up, it will start to spill out into the biggest organ on your body, which is your skin. Any problems you might have in your colon will start to show up in your skin first. If your body has any toxins that it is unable to get rid of, then these toxins will build up in your fat cells, leading to inflammation over the area with the real problem; it is almost like an arrow pointing to the problem.

You can start your detox here by cleaning out the skin. An obvious method is to learn how to sweat. Aerobic exercise is best for increasing oxygen usage and pushing fluids through the skin. Sweating opens up the pores, flushing them out and clearing away the excess toxins coming out from your colon.

Far Infrared Sauna

Our body absorbs 4-14 microns of the sun's wavelength that causes the water molecules of our bodies to pulsate and break down to small molecules thus allowing easy entry into the cells. These clusters of water molecules that keep your DNA from falling apart surround your DNA. There is a release of endothelial nitric oxide that allows your capillaries to dilate, increasing tissue oxygenation and opening the skin pores without overusing the liver detox pathway. The Far Infrared Sauna is one of the best ways to eliminate heavy metals, pesticides, and environmental chemicals from our bodies. You also tend to release weight by speeding up the metabolism and regenerate the beauty of your skin. It is also very relaxing to the mind, not to mention that we often release emotions while in the sauna. It is one of my favorite devices.

Then we come to the colon itself. Half of the population has low stomach acid, which makes it difficult for the stomach to properly digest and break down proteins. As a result, the stomach creates additional compounds to do so, which get absorbed into the small intestine, triggering a host of reactions. People with low stomach acid can get migraines, sinus problems, become fat deficient, Vitamin B12 deficient, and have problems absorbing iron, and so on. Low stomach acid is like clogging the pipes in your house and backing up the sewers. Water will build up as a result, altering the acidity of the body, which can cause the calcium in the bones to break down and start depositing all over the body. Additionally, since the body is not fully digesting the food, it starts to build up in the colon and just rots there, producing toxins and excessive bacterial growth. Ever seen a house where there is mold growing on the walls? Have you seen how it affects the health of everyone living there? A dirty colon is like that. The colon really is a garbage dump. Some people can lose 25 pounds if they just flush their colon of all this old debris. The simplest way to do this is just drink a lot of water, preferably non-chlorinated and non-fluoridated to promote better absorption. The water will hydrate your body enough to allow it to get rid of the old stool. Drink about half your body weight in ounces throughout each day to keep things moving. We also use rectal ozone insufflation that helps eliminate the "bugs" including bacteria, viruses, and parasites. Rectal ozone, some expert say, is as good as intravenous ozone treatment with stimulating of the immune system. Two other procedures we use in late stage patients are coffee enema and/or wheat grass implants. Our healthy clients can also use this procedure for overall health bi-yearly. These procedures dilate the portal bed and release large amounts of antioxidants into the system.

Another issue with the colon is stress. Emotional issues, resentment, anger, all that stuff that angry people hold in will cramp your colon as well. Release the pent up emotions and you will also release your bowels. If the stool is hard and difficult to empty, lay off the coffee and coke. Another problem is artificial sweeteners; they can destroy good bacterial flora by half, which is bad for nutrient absorption. Some medications can also reduce beneficial bacterial flora, and as if that was not bad enough, such medications often use a bit of artificial sweeteners to add flavor. Any type of liquid can contain artificial sweeteners, be it colas or medications. So watch those labels.

When one of my patients first came to see me, the doctors had her scheduled for knee replacement surgery. I took her off artificial sweeteners and the next day she was well. Eight years later and still no knee surgery. A good healthy diet and plenty of water will go a long way to curing your ailments.

There are other ways to help the colon as well. One is a colon massage, a simple massage from above the appendix area, descending down to the rectal area. You can squat down on the ground for a bit to encourage a bowel movement. Honey and lemon in hot water is also good for getting things moving. The key, though, is to have enough acid in your gut and keep the right bacterial flora populating your gut.

Oral swishes are another method. Swish some coconut oil or sesame oil around in your mouth for five minutes then spit it out. Afterwards drink some water, rinse it out, repeatedly until it comes out clear. You are cleaning out toxins as well as your supporting your teeth.

Oh, and by the way, there is a practical use for that cola drink. Pour it into your toilet bowl and let it sit there for about an hour. It is great for getting it sparkly clean!

3. Detoxing the Lymph System

The lymph system is where the leftovers from the blood vessels end up, bacteria, bits of leftover protein, debris of all kinds. It is like the people in the house, making sure things stay organized, prioritized, cleaned out before the body recirculates it back into the blood stream. Like your mother, mopping up the floor after you tracked your muddy feet across it. If you are suffering from excess weight, pain such as headaches, arthritis, bursitis, tendonitis, slow metabolism or immune system with difficulty in overcoming infections or trauma, you just may be dealing with a clogged lymphatic system.

One of the best ways to get your lymph moving is by exercising. My favorite way of doing this is the rebounder; just jumping up and down on it 5 to 10 minutes a day can make a big difference. Getting the lymph to flow will clean out the lymph nodes and keep them properly functioning. A good lymph system will keep the white blood cells circulating, prevent fat buildup, and helps keep everything moving along. There are many other ways such as deep breathing exercising, chi machines, PEMF, foot massagers, reflexology, dry skin brushing, hot and cold contrast baths (which are incredible) and, of course, having a massage about every three to six months.

4. Detoxing The Lungs

The lungs are the air conditioning of your house. Your body needs proper ventilation, because oxygen is key to your entire metabolism. The key to clean lungs is breathing clean air. If the air in your house is stagnant, filled with particulate matter, and possibly fungal buildup, then you need to change the clogged filters of your air conditioner, or get an air purifier. Having plants around the house is also a good and natural way to keep the air clean.

Exercise is a great way to clean out the lungs. It is akin to cleaning the air filters on your home's A/C intake. Another way to clean the lungs is the hydrogen peroxide food grade heavily diluted nasal puffer...but only under a physician's supervision. Yet another method is drinking a glass of water with a pinch of sea salt. This will act as a natural antihistamine, helping the respiratory system as well as reducing the amount of histamine exposure. Another natural antihistamine that is good for the lungs is Vitamin C. Finally, saunas and steam rooms will clear up the lungs as well.

Of course, you should avoid anything that clogs up the lungs. Smoking is at the top of the list; besides inhaling smoke and carcinogens, you are also inhaling radium, which is radioactive and hence notoriously difficult to get rid of.

Emotions can also end up affecting your lungs. As you feel, so does your house look. If you are depressed, you do not clean the house, which leads to all sorts of air pollutants, which you breathe in, thus affecting your energy and health, which in turn makes you feel even worse. Take a serious look at your emotional state and see how it is affecting your house, car, and general environment.

Anything that exercises the lungs is beneficial; keep the air moving and you will keep things cleaned out. This could be normal exercising or sports, but also playing a harmonica, bugle, singing, breathing exercises, or anything at all that works the lungs.

5. Detoxify Your Blood

Blood is the gas and water of the house of your body. Keeping it clean and pure is very important, but also very easy. By the time you have gone about cleaning your colon, bladder, lymph, and lungs, you have already done the job of cleaning out your blood supply. Just make sure that you are drinking the best quality water possible.

6. Detoxify Your Nervous System

The nervous system is the telephone system of your house. Its function is to keep everything communicating with everything else, which makes it of prime importance. Faulty lines of communication can cause a host of problems.

Heavy metals are a big issue with the nervous system, particularly Mercury. Mercury easily blocks the tubulins I mentioned earlier that transmit light. The amount of Mercury found in one cheap dental filling is enough to cause a problem. Some products from China, like tuna and swordfish, also contain Mercury. Mercury can cross the blood-brain barrier, causing such problems as Alzheimer's disease, Parkinson's disease, Multiple Sclerosis, and so on.

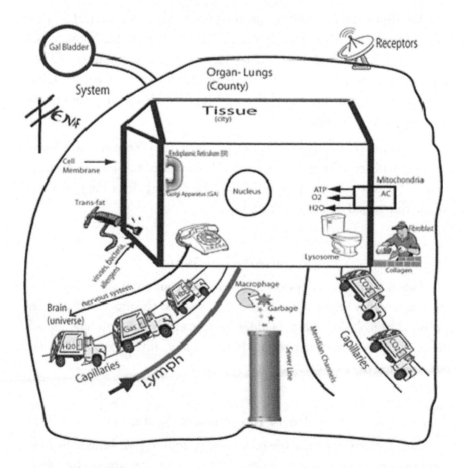

Getting rid of these heavy metals is not easy, but it is possible. I use laser energy detoxification, which can have dramatic effects, but chelation agents such as iodine also work, as does taking DMSA orally, which also helps with chelation. Simpler ways of ridding yourself of heavy metals, like Mercury, are supplements such as chlorella, spirulina, and cilantro. Chlorella is algae and, like the others, it cannot hurt you. Chlorella works by latching onto the heavy metal particles and ushering them out of the body. Once the body clears itself of these heavy metal toxins, the nervous system can repair itself. Choline is a supplement that that will actually rebuild your nervous system, like rewiring your house.

Once your body clears itself of such heavy metals as Mercury and its ilk, remarkable things can happen.

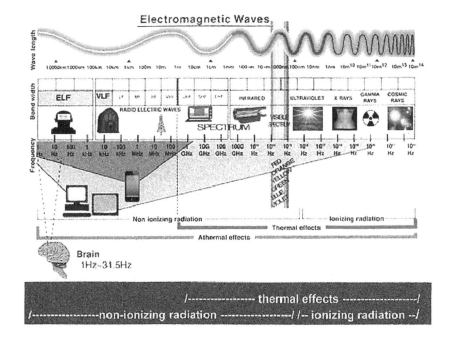

Electromagnetic Frequency Toxicity

WiFi, cell phones, and cell phone towers pollute our environment with electromagnetic waves. Cell phones can cause a certain amount of heat induction into the skull, but even more significant is the carrier wave of the signal, the part carrying the information. This heat induction can cause issues in the connections between the cells in your body, causing some damage, and in the case of having a cell phone by your head, can give you headaches. It is important that you shield your cell phone and other appliances. Putting ear buds into your ears will actually increase the problem by about 300%. Just recently in Lyon, France, the International Agency for Research on Cancer classified cell phones as possible carcinogenic agents, putting them in the same category as the pesticide DDT, gasoline engine exhaust, and coffee.

Electromagnetic Frequency (EMF) toxicity in a person is like living in a house next to the person with the shortwave radio; you will get interference on every television set in your house until you find a way of shielding against it.

Electromagnetic radiation from other sources, though, can be more of a problem. One extreme method would be to build a canopy over your bed for radiation shielding, but that is not what I do. I do a lot of prayer to ensure my belief system is healthy, because belief can have tremendous power. Believe in your heart that God is your protection and he will be.

Other ways of protecting yourself is to keep your cell phone away from your heart and reproductive organ. The best place I put mine is on my desk no less than about four feet from me. If someone calls you on the cell phone and if you know it is going to take more than 3 minutes to answer their questions, then politely tell them you will call them on a land line. If you are driving, then get outside the car because the EMFs are bouncing all over the inside of the car. If you cannot leave the car (like if you are driving down the freeway) then roll down your window and place the phone on speaker. If the strength is low, do not answer your phone, and if it drops low while on a call, then just hang up and call them back when the signal is better. The brain is a terrible thing to fry, so these are my humble suggestions for keeping it cool.

Please do not allow young children to use a cell phone. Their skulls are much thinner and the thermal frequency and the carrier waves transmit even deeper. They should only use the cell phone if there is an emergency that requires its use.

Avoid using smart meters and take necessary precautions by not having one installed. They are not too "smart" to have on your home or around you. They are only smart for the industry and the people who make money off collecting data about you and your family. To check the EMF, simply purchase a gauss meter and get within 20 feet of the smart meter. Then see how much continuous electromagnetic radiation with the wifi and pulsatile radiation interacts with the smart meter. Then stand in front of the gauss meter and see how much your body absorbs. The wall will not absorb it but your body will absorb close to 100%. Your body's intelligent design never intended you to be dealing with this amount of EMF.

Also, throw away your alarm clock and cordless phones. And if you have a cordless phone, do not have the base near your sleeping area.

Homes should have no compact fluorescent lights in their environment. They require a large amount of mercury to form the ultraviolet spectrum wavelength. This is quite damaging, especially for people who have autoimmune issues such as skin problems, lupus, diabetes, rheumatoid, etc. I helped one gentleman who worked on an oil rig whose blood sugar was normal when on the ocean, but when back at home it would go to 300 and he would have to take 60 units of insulin. I asked him if he had any CFL's in his home and he confirmed that he had them all over the house. I told him to replace the fluorescent bulbs in his living area with incandescent bulbs. He did. As a result he no longer had to take insulin. There are better options such as LED bulbs. They last longer, but they are slightly more expensive. Another option is just to use the regular old light bulbs... as long as they are still on the market.

7. General Detoxifying

For detoxifying in general, you just need to look at your diet. I recommend juicing: fruits, vegetables, mix it up with some almond milk, maybe some chia seed to increase the fiber. Juice it up with a bit of soluble fiber, and you are good to go. If you are gluten intolerant, then you can use millet and brown rice. You can even throw an egg in there for more protein; eggs are very healthy.

Mix your own brew of detoxifying raw foods together and have a deep swig once a day. Your body will love you for it.

The Case Of Ivllon Holt Zachary

I am a registered nurse. In 1996, I had a faulty heat exchanger unit that gave me a chronic exposure to low levels of carbon monoxide. I became very ill, had a lowered immune system, and by September of 1999, had flu-like symptoms, could not get well, was septic, had a staff infection, was bed bound, and could not get up from my wheelchair. My doctors declared me permanently disabled and said I had less than 5 years to live. I was taking all kinds of medications that were toxic to my liver.

By the time I saw Dr. Lucky in 2000, I'd been on chemo for 6½ years, had a pain pump in me, had arthritis, fibromialgia, pneumonia every few months, was on oxygen every day, walked with a shuffled gait, was on 30 medications, and had to have someone else drive. I had poor circulation in both legs, my hands were swollen closed, carpal tunnel in both hands, fibrosis in both lungs, sepsis, saw 10 doctors a month, and despite the valium, I was still in pain. I was an invalid, unable to walk more than 10 or 12 feet, and was told I would not have lived more than 5 years because of the damage to my liver from the drugs given to me.

*Dr. Lucky started me on nutrients, and then used his laser light machine, bioenergy therapy, the Ondamed machine, and used prayer and positive motivation. I was given sentences to say on a daily basis, like **"I choose to be well."***

There were certain emotional issues I had in the past; abandonment, loss, and traumatic events in my life. Dr. Lucky helped me deal with all this. He told me that my younger sister and I were very close, and that both of us were close to our dad, which was amazing because it was true! I hadn't told him a thing! As a kid, our mother would put castor oil in our orange juice, which made me gag, but forced me to drink thinking it was healthy; that later made it difficult for me to take liquid meds. Dr. Lucky helped me to understand that my mom meant the best and to not resent her; this helped me to resolve my emotional issues that helped in curing me. Dr. Lucky says that we are all con-nected through energy, connected spiritually, so it is a good thing for my family to see my improvement for their sake as well.

I am now pain free, can run with no help, am down to 1 or 2 meds, and use no other doctors or specialists, and it's been more than 5 years. I refer my friends to him now.

The Doctor's Notes:

She was referred to us by a lady who was a relative of another patient of mine. Doctors diagnosed her with crippling Rheumatoid Arthritis. The doctors were using a double Remicade dosage that costs about $5000 per month and not seeing results. It took about a month of prayer and nutrients and she was back to working full time.

Ivllon is an amazing young lady with an amazing testimony of what God did in her life. She could write a book and it would take 100 pages alone just to summarize what happened. One major event occurred about the third visit. She was sitting in the chair, and I was observing her fingers and she told me her fingers popped. I said *"So, what?."* She then stated she had not done that for twenty years. I asked her to see what she could do with her hand, so she closed her hand and I almost passed out. At our first meeting I could not even examine her hands due to the swelling, much less check to see how strong she was.

She is now a surrogate to other people and has no issues testing herself. Ivllon has been such an angel and is probably responsible for hundreds of new patients coming to me from throughout the United States and around the world. A new update on Ivllon, about two years ago she kite surfed the Gulf of Mexico with her grandson and the boat stopped and she and grandson fell to the water. The boat dragged her under four feet of water for about 40 feet. Her grandson could not swim and she had to save him. The person who tried to rescue them froze and she had to save him as well. Can you imagine a person who was in a wheelchair with severe crippling Rheumatoid Arthritis on a pain pump about 10 years earlier saving people from drowning in the shark infested waters of the Gulf of Mexico. God is so Good!

The Case Of Sophia Culpepper,
Daughter of Brandy and Russel

⋘◄•►⋙

Sophia was 11 months old and very sick. She was projectile vomiting, 20 to 30 times a day, had a life-threatening allergy to milk, and was on a special prescription formula that costs $80 a can. I had taken her to specialists, hospitals, and no one knew what to do.

I had heard of Dr. Lucky through my pastor and decided to give him a try. He started out with prayer and put her on supplements; Vitamin B6, aloe, and water. He then questioned me about her, and asked if she had had any vaccinations. Of course she had, and Dr. Lucky said her vaccinations were causing autoimmune diseases. (He did not know that she had been medically documented with autoimmune diseases.) He recommended that we give her no more vaccinations.

My daughter stopped vomiting the first day I brought her in to see Dr. Lucky. Now, some four months since, has still not vomited. She could never tolerate proteins before, but now she has scrambled eggs for breakfast. She still has some problems with milk, but no more vomiting it back out.

When she was first vaccinated, there was a white spot on her leg; they said it would eventually take over her entire body and make her an albino. Well, since seeing Dr. Lucky, it has stopped growing, and we have hopes that it will be entirely healed as well.

Dr. Lucky is intelligent, with a matter-of-fact attitude. Sophia's quality of life has greatly improved and she is now doing really well.

The Doctor's Notes:

Sophia is an eleven- month young white female, here for nutritional counseling and evaluation. Her mother had some complications with pregnancy, and the child had severe projectile vomiting 20-30 times per day that began with the first bottle feed. Her doctor prescribed Reglan for both the mother and the child, without much success. Doctor told her the bottle was equal to breast feeding, so they started her on Similac Advance, which she vomited, and diagnosed her with a milk allergy and rice allergy. The young patient almost died, turned blue after having milk. Two weeks ago with GERD, but later pH testing revealed no GERD. She received her Hepatitis vaccine, as well as a long list of vaccines prior to passing blood, and the doctor diagnosed her with allergic colitis at around two months of age, as well as protein intolerance. She would vomit after getting shots at 6 and 8 months, "throwing up her guts". Then three weeks ago, after the flu shot, she had a fever and eczema on her faced erupted. She was failing to thrive and had developed a large patch of vitiligo on her legs.

An energetic test revealed a severe stomach imbalance affecting the brain stem, nervous system, lymphatic, and cardiovascular system, as well as having a virus and uterus imbalance. She was definitely sensitive to milk and gluten, and her heart point was very elevated without primary heart being an issue. Vaccinations often contain Casein products. Therefore, due to the parallel to the shots, I do not recommend them.

I discussed with the mother that I am not a pediatrician, but with the vitiligo presenting following a shot on the masculine side of the body, another shot could be dangerous. Because she was not able to have a shot soon, I told the family that we would see how she did when the body is detoxed. We used Laser Energy Detoxification (LED) on the child, with vaccination, heavy metal, and sucralose, and I discussed with the mother any emotional issues in the family. We had one follow-up call a couple of days later; Sophia was better, but I have not heard from them since.

" Diseases are to be diagnosed andprevented via energy field assessment. "

-George Crile MD Sr.

Chapter SIX

7 Incredible Technological Breakthroughs Your Doctor Hates

Chemicals and toxins are the basis for medical technology, which the body has great difficulty processing. There are many other technologies for diagnosis and healing that are not based on toxic pharmaceuticals. In this chapter, we are going to cover seven of my favorites; alternatives that I employ in my own clinic almost every day. George Crile Sr., founder of the Cleveland Clinic, said it well, "Diseases are to be diagnosed and prevented by energy field assessment!"

1. The Ondamed

Several scanning technologies operate within a frequency range that actually creates havoc for your body. The Ondamed is a Class 2 Biofeedback Device in the category of neurology, approved for use as a noninvasive secondary therapeutic device. It allows you to scan the body at different frequencies, much like tuning a radio; if you are at the right frequency, then you get a clear and crisp sound on the radio. We scan over the body and feel for a pulse. If there is a disturbance in your electrical system, then you will get a convergence of a wave, the amplitude of the wave increasing so that you will feel a slight bump, indicating a disturbance…that something is not right. It allows you actually to feel the location of the problem. It is similar to a sonar for the body.

More than that though, the Ondamed then allows you to dial in a particular frequency that will actually neutralize or balance that disturbance in the body. This is one of the most powerful devices that I have come across in my life and is the number one device on my list.

Imbalances cause illness and the aging process. Metabolic processes produce leftovers called free radicals, which go around trying to interact with anything with which they come in contact, including your DNA. This activity throws the body out of balance, so it tries to heal itself. Too much healing is also not a good thing. In fact, some so-called cancers are essentially the healing process run amok. Both situations lead to imbalance and the outcome is disease, which creates even more of an imbalance, and so on. It is a vicious cycle that becomes very damaging, so we need to achieve a balance for the body.

There are drugs that reduce inflammation, but inflammation is the body's way to heal, so burying that is also not a good thing. The Ondamed balances the frequencies of the tissues that are imbalanced with a counter frequency of its own. A waveform is composed of crests and troughs; the crests are the problem areas. The Ondamed counters that with a waveform that matches troughs to these crests, leveling everything out and bringing balance back to the problem area. It balances out the energy field of the body, which is a very powerful technique.

Picture the ocean, the wave coming in at the beach. If one wave happens to go in at the same time as the previous one is pulling back out, then the first is a crest while the older one is a trough. They will cancel and the crest of the new wave will not be as big. If a wave comes in and right behind it is another new wave, then if they collide their crests will add, creating a single larger wave.

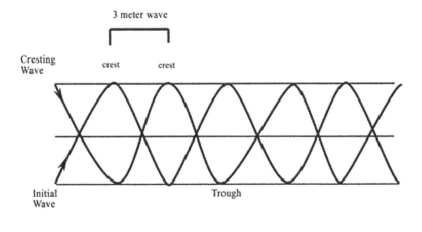

Frequency $= f = c/\lambda = (3 \times 10^8 \text{ m/s}) / 3m = 10^8$ cycles/sec

Speed of Light $= c = 3 \times 10^8$ m/s

Wavelength $= \lambda$ In bio-energetic medicine we are attempting to cancel the aberrant wave patterns by using a canceling waves and promoting health and wellness. Everything including bacteria, virus, parasites, words, thoughts, cells, organs, galaxies etc vibrates at a certain frequency. We need balancing not destruction in our universe today.

This is essentially the process that occurs with the Ondamed. Einstein's famous formula states that Energy equals Mass times the Speed of Light squared, which is saying that all matter is energy, and energy is light. We are measuring light and manipulating the light field of the human body.

Some people would call this a placebo effect, claiming that the effect directly correlates to the intent. In reality, since the effect relates to intent (your intent to heal), it does have a measurable effect on the body. There is a classic experiment in Quantum Mechanics known as the double-slit experiment. First, a person fires a beam of electrons through a slit onto a screen beyond it. This experiment results in the image on the screen looking like a fan with decreasing uniformly as you move farther away from the center. This pattern is what one would expect for particles. Then, the person fires a beam of electrons through two slits, one next to the other. Now you notice bands of interference, so it appears to be waves instead of particles. In an effort to explain this, they then put in an observer whose job was to concentrate on what he wanted the outcome to be—a particle or a wave. They found that the observer's desired intent altered the resultant pattern. The observer's intent determines the so-called placebo effect. A real measurable effect related to the way light behaves.

Energy is light, and just as light is a source of life and energy for plants, researchers are finding that our bodies have a bit of light in them as well. Research has scientifically proven that we generate our own faint light field, our glow rising and falling over the course of the day. This field of light emission connects our entire body, pulls every cell in our bodies together and ties them one to another. This is the basis for the likes of acupuncture, where a tiny pressure in one spot transmits to other parts of the body within seconds by an effect known as the piezoelectric effect, where the body converts pressure into electricity.

The Ondamed makes use of all this, tweaking specific spots in our overall electric field which then pass these changes onto the organs and tissues from which they emanate.

2. The Zyto

Another feedback device is the Zyto. This one is a bit difficult to understand. Basically, it reads the digital frequency of a substance. Without getting too heavy into the Quantum Physics of it, the Zyto looks at what is measured and tells you the frequency the substance is emanating. Then it gives you a comparison of how far the reading is from normal. It gives a direct measure of the stresses put upon the body. I then use that information to make remedies.

I first interview the patient, take their history, and listen to their bodies to get a general idea of where the problem lies. I then use the Zyto to pinpoint things more precisely. The Zyto will allow me to find a counter-frequency, which I then imprint into a solution for the patient to drink. I have had patients for which the curative results occurred within minutes.

I use the Zyto to see if I am missing anything. Zyto can test for about twenty to thirty thousand different items in a manner of five or six minutes. It allows me to read the energy patterns of the human body and gives me an idea of which therapeutic direction to take.

I once treated a young lady in her 20's who was having difficulty with her marriage due to fatigue, bloating, palpitations, and irritability, not to mention she was pretty hateful to her husband and family. I scanned her and found out that her hormones were all over the place. I placed her on the Zyto for a historical reading of her body, and that indicated an imbalance in DHEA, estrogen, and progesterone. We imprinted the homeopathic frequencies and had great results. Her husband, who did not want her to come see me in the first place, called me to let me know how much he appreciated my treating his wife.

3. The Evox

This one has to do with voice mapping, which is reading what a person says. Evox facilitates perception reframing, which is a technique that gives us a different way of seeing circumstances and opportunities, challenges or relationships. I use this in instances when someone comes to the clinic with an issue that is hard to deal with and we are having trouble identifying where it is coming from. This device allows us to look at the emotional imprint of the patient. This is very helpful because it is all about the patient, not the "other person." At first, they may think it is about the other person, but this device allows the patient to see that this is really just the distorted perception of an event or situation. If the Evox program balances out the emotional disturbance, then the body will take it from there and improve things.

We simply talk to the patient, talk about the pain, and then do a map. If the map shows a pattern of stagnation, then we have a problem. We then need to get the patient to see what is stuck to make it disappear to correct it. It is like being unable to improve your golf game because subconsciously you think that you are a loser and bad golfer and that interferes with playing the game. Eliminate the distorted belief pattern and the emotions will proceed into balance.

Evox has a wide range of applications including addictions, self-improvement, etc. You just need to talk about it, and then the machine gives you the feedback that you need to overcome it.

A 65-year young lady came to see us who had severe skin issues, thought to be psoriasis by multiple physicians. They had treated her with steroids, all kinds of topicals, and lymphatic drainage techniques. The doctors also had treated her with the Ondamed, Zyto, phototherapy, essential oils, and homeopathics, but had no success. Plaque was all over her arms, upper and lower legs, as well as her neck. We placed her on the Evox and did a voice mapping of her husband and daughter, and then had her drink the imprinted water for 24 hours. Except for a small amount on her right wrist, the rash completely disappeared! The emotion behind the skin was separated out, after which healing began. The skin is our integrity, our boundary. We have all heard people described as tough skinned or thin skinned, and this old saying can literally apply as a connection between our emotions and some skin conditions.

4. Micro-current Therapy

When we go through any type of trauma, the electrical potential of the cell changes. In a healthy person, the electrical potential of the average cell runs about -70 millivolts, but when you have a disease, this number starts to decrease. If you get to around -40, you are close to death. At -20, the cell is essentially frozen, meaning nothing going in or coming out. Micro-current therapy is a way of giving a small current over a very short duration, like a minute or two, and in rare instances as much as five minutes.

Trauma induces an entry current around the area, and when you are sick, it becomes dense and nothing can penetrate the tissue. Electricity goes from a higher resistance to a lower resistance, and so tries to go around it. By giving these small micro-currents, we then neutralize that effect and restore the flow around where the traumatic current is taking place. Research shows that small electrical charges may be helpful in initiating and perpetuating the numerous electrical chemical reactions that allow for healing to manifest itself. There is a speculation that micro-current works to decrease pain by reducing its cause and altering the electrical activity of the surrounding tissue. This process increases a cell's energy production by three to five folds, opens up the channels so nutrients can get through, and instantaneously starts boosting protein synthesis and production.

When someone has clogged up systems and the lymphatic system is not working well, then I use micro-current or the Ondamed to put movement into the tissue. This allows the lymphatic system to move and clean out the system, providing significant detoxification. It also works with something called noceo-receptors in the blood vessels, improving circulation that can fix other problems you did not even know you had. I have worked on people's toes and all of a sudden their frozen shoulder that they have had for 20 years opens up and they can now move it without any restrictions whatsoever! This is because the body is 100% connected, so when you use these devices, you can have dramatic changes anywhere in the body.

A young lady in her 70's came in with what she called a migraine headache for two straight days without relief. She was obviously very tired when I saw her. We took about 5 minutes and did micro-current using the temple point bilaterally and the headache went away instantly. She wrote to me and told me the last time she had to go to a hospital, she had spent $500 for a shot and the headache returned two hours later. This time it went away and stayed away.

5. Laser Energy Detoxification (LED)

LED is a noninvasive method that lacks approval by the FDA, so using it is totally up to the patient. Any risk is exceedingly low with this procedure.

Each of us has numerous points in our bodies that produce light, some near the surface, and others that are very deep within, such as the organs. This therapy works like acupressure on these points within the body. Often, we will incorporate this device with the Zyto, because we can make remedies of balance with the Zyto, and then take those reme-dies and sweep over the body with a laser. Incredible things can happen in seconds with this process. I have used this to treat a myriad of condi-tions in our clinic, but we do not charge for it because it takes a total of about 5 seconds. We know that organisms like bacteria, viruses, and par-asites vibrate at certain frequencies, so LED can balance these frequen-cies as well. When you sweep with the laser, you can dislodge all kinds of issues, even issues of the emotional kind.

We have seen this help balance hormones. People who had devel-oped a resistance to insulin have had their issues reversed. Some of my clients who had taken insulin for years do not even need to take it any-more. We have seen clients reduce their need for medicine to a minimum. I am not necessarily against medicine, just inefficient usage. I use the LED in order to balance the whole body at once and not just specific spots. That goes a long way toward curing and detoxing the body.

A 40 something young female came in with severe bilateral allergic conjunctival involvement. She could not stop rubbing her eyes. I went outside, obtained some pollen off my car and placed the pollen in a vial. I then swept over her eyes and adrenal glands and the irritation went away bilaterally in about two minutes.

I also treated a young lady in her 60's who was not able to see out of her left eye, had a visual acuity of 20/200, and bleeding behind the eye. The doctor felt she needed surgery within two weeks. We evaluated her and found weakness in the left eye as well as splenic weakness, indicating a bleeding wound. We used phototherapy, LED, and started her on V-Statin nutritional supplements. Within two weeks, she returned to the doctor and her vision had improved to 20/50 with no bleeding. As of this writing, it has been about one year and she believes her vision is now normal. She did not require surgery. Thank you, God!

6. Ancestral Mapping

Now we get to the one of the very unconventional techniques that we use. I developed this technique myself. I call it ancestral mapping, and every patient that walks in the door receives this benefit.

People are linked to the people in their past. The connection is so close that they have similar conditions and even die in similar ways as their ancestors. I have found the link correlates to how close they were to their predecessors. This is not genetics. It is epigenetics! The goal is to uncover the root issue. What is causing their system to clog up? What is the emotional linkage? The link focuses on the similar emotions that you or your ancestors have had. We evaluate those emotions, allowing the left side of our brain to uncover what is there.

The right side of the brain controls the left side of the body, while the left side of the brain controls the right side of the body. The right side of the brain is creative and musical. Right side of the brain focuses on finding solutions to our problems. It is instantaneous and spontaneous. It does not have to make any sense, and most of the time it does not.

The left side of the brain, however, focuses on linear, logical, concrete thinking. The right side of the brain is the present side of the brain, while the left side reacts to fear, anxiety, stress, guilt, and shame. True healing change occurs in the Present, so we help disconnect from the Past in order to affect change. I have some techniques that I use to discover the errant beliefs and in literally seconds work on correcting those beliefs. The troubling beliefs are most often not theirs in the first place.

When someone recognizes that a belief is not theirs and can clearly see the exact pattern and where everything is coming from, it enables them to have a tremendous shift into the Present. Often, the things we are dealing with are events that happened in the past. But our Present is determined by what is happening right now, what our ideas are right now, not "back then." We help our clients to stop trying to solve a problem in the Past, focus on the Present, and move on with their lives. As soon as they do this, transformation of lives occur.

If someone holds resentment, unforgiveness, or anger towards another person, they also hold themselves in bondage with that person until that chain is broken. Your body will hold that kernel of anger and resentment, tie it up into a knot, and put it somewhere in your body. It could show up as a pain in the stomach, a problem in the back, or any number of things. This is an important therapy because it deals with the root issue of the emotion so much faster and can completely remove the need for medications and their side effects. All that is required is a desire for healing, and the good news is that your body already wants to be healed. Ancestral Mapping helps you find a way through what is holding you back.

Heart Math

Whereas Ancestral Mapping clears you into the present moment, Heart Math procedure basis is on the autonomic nervous system, which is subconscious. It looks at the heart and its connection to the brain, to find what is hiding and trying to prevent us from finding the real problem.

If your body is balanced, it is harmonious with the sympathetic nervous system. This is that part of the nervous system that triggers the flight response and the stress response of the human body. This technique allows you to breathe and also help you get into the present moment. Focus on an emotional stimulus about a particular situation and just feel the heart focus and you will sense that your body gets into a rhythm with your heart and your nervous system; that is coherent. When your mind is chaotic and thinking too fast, then it is incoherent. This often occurs when the heart has made the brain toxic and the brain simply cannot take anymore, so it closes the gate between the sympathetic and parasympathetic nervous system. By reducing the stress pattern, the brain can once again open up the gate and heal the body according to its design. We use heart math to evaluate people to see if their body is "in the mood" to heal. If it is not in the mood, we employ these procedures to get them back into some coherency.

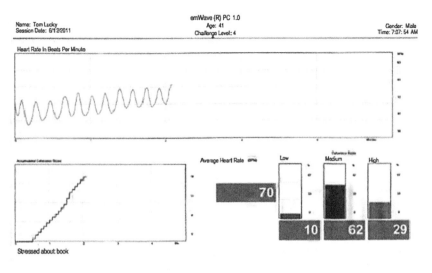

Heart math uses the heart rate variability device and indicates changes in the heart rate. It reveals how well the heart is dealing with stress. A higher number on the scale indicates you are dealing better with stress. Personally, I started out with two, but now I am up to a four, which is the highest. Even when I broke my neck and fractured four ribs, I was able to keep myself in a place of peace and calm.The heart can be full of fear, so we help people take the emotion of love and put it back into the heart. That really is foundational to our clinic's purpose and passion. My clinic is all about the heart: hope, love, choices.

There are devices you can purchase that will help your body get into coherence. When you get angry about something and your day is not going right, this exercise will show you a way out. If you do some breathing and work with it, get your heart and brain back in training, you will feel a tremendous amount of improvement. Your heart is the best and largest electromagnetic field in the human body; it emanates from your body to influence people around you.

A success story using heart math is that of a 65-year young man with a known history of reoccurring atrial fibrillation, which constantly got him hospitalized. He came in with atrial fibrillation and a heart rate in the

140 range, but was hemodynamically stable. I placed him on the monitor and hooked him up to the heart rate variability device. I disclosed to him that someone had been in his territory and that he was trying to heal from that. His wife stated they knew who it was and I asked him to think about that same man as a child coming into the world innocent with loving parents. Immediately when he thought about this person in this alternative context, his heart went into normal rhythm and became coherent. His heart has not been out of rhythm since, which was two years ago.

Sometimes it only takes one visit. Other times, it takes more. I can never tell, so I tell patients that I cannot guarantee. It is all up to the body and how the body wants to use the information and how much they desire to get well. People usually see a positive effect in their lives within a month, sometimes instantaneously. If the improvement is dramatic enough, I do not even recommend they come back.

The Herring rule definition is the body heals from the top of your head to the bottom of your feet, from the inside to outside. The way God designed the body to heal. People diagnosed with asthma typically have a skin irritation or inflammation at birth; the asthma actually comes later. When their asthma disappears, the skin rash comes back; the body is healing in reverse fashion, and that is how you know when your body is actually improving. Keep in mind that when you start going through these cleansings, the worst thing you can do is to see medical doctors who do not understand the holistic process, because they will prescribe antibiotics and/or steroids to treat the current condition, instead of looking at the overall process.

7. Pulse Electromagnetic Frequency Device (PEMF)

According to NASA reports, the earth's magnetic field is collapsing rapidly. Experts believe that the earth's EMF has dropped from nearly 30 Gauss at the time of the dinosaurs to 0.3 Gauss today. Because we humans have a substance in our pineal gland called magnetite (as most animals do) to help with our homing, we are directly affected by the magnetic field of the earth. So what is the problem with magnetic field deficiency, you ask? (1) Increase acidosis (2) Thickened blood that increases the risk of stroke and heart attack (3) Decreased oxygen getting to the cells, (4) Increased toxicity caused by the cells' compromised ability to move healthy things into the cells and rid the cells of unhealthy things that are damaging to the body. This essentially causes a stagnant pond (fermentation effect) which eventually leads to death, due to severe lymphatic congestion. (5) Decreased energy, a.k.a. fatigue.

The cell is like a battery. The cell membrane stores voltage and capacitance. It is an insulator and promotes the integrity of the cell, as discussed in a previous chapter. The Voltage potential is usually around -70 mv range which is considered a healthy cell, with more an-ions on the inside and more cat-ions on the outside. We start experiencing degeneration at about -40 mv and when we have "so called" cancer dedifferentiation, it is around -20 mv and the cell is drowning in all its toxic milieu.

PEMF allows for the reversal of these processes by using short bursts of electromagnetic energy pulses that promote excitation of atoms, resulting in a magnetic field, which literally can shake fragile (unhealthy) cells apart. Then the body's cleaning crews (macrophages) are activated, it is able to digest and reuse whatever parts it can, while eliminating the parts that are unhealthy to the cell by a process called Autophagy. This same pulse will strengthen healthy cell membranes and allow for changes in trans-membrane potential, thus increasing permeability and allowing selective increased electron flux by activating ATP pump on the cell membranes. What does all this mean?

1. Oxygenation increases by about 200% to the cells.
2. Because of the increased negative charge on the membranes, they now repel themselves, which allows more freedom of movement and alkalinity of the tissues.
3. With increased alkalinity, there is decreased inflammation and swelling.
4. Increased ability with pumps working due to increased energy provided by the ATP from mitochondria excitation to get the nutrients in and the toxic waste out.

The case of D.W

This young man came in to see me with acute blindness of his left eye. We placed him on the PEMF device and by the next visit he could see light in his peripheral vision. But he was also very excited about his right shoulder in which he had had a rotator cuff tear for 20 years, which led to a frozen shoulder. After the initial treatment, he had full range of motion. I saw him about 6 months later and he still had full range of motion in the shoulder.

Another gentleman had severe congestive cardiomyopathy with EF of 20% and taking maximum therapy with a pharmaceutical bill around $1,500 dollars per month. He was short of breath and could only walk about 20 feet without having to sit down for several minutes before continuing. He had been sleeping in a chair because of the fluid suffocating him at night. We used diet modification, emotional counseling, present techniques, started him on about $150 worth of supplements including D-Ribose, Magnesium, L Carnitine, Glyconutrient Powder, Vortex water, and Coenzyme Q 10 and PQQ complex along with PEMF treatments. Within two weeks, he was only taking 3 pharmaceutical medications and had lost 30 pounds of fluid. He had discontinued the diuretics medication and was walking 2 miles per day without shortness of breath. He was sleeping in his bed and after 6 months, he was using his push lawn mower to mow his large lawn in 90-degree heat. To God be all the glory for this man's recovery. And I know much of the effectiveness of his treatment was due to the effect the PEMF has on stem cells and its ability to increase growth factors, endorphins, and hormones in the body. PEMF has shown to increase the length of telomeres on the ends of chromosomes of our DNA, which is correlated to our life span.

PEMF is also very good for healthy people, sports enthusiasts, and weight release because it increases adiponectin. Low levels of adiponectin are associated with increased insulin resistance and, in my opinion, "so called" cancer is nothing more than severe insulin resistance. This is why a ketogenic diet tends to have such a positive curative effect.

The Case Of Ted Maxie
As Told By Ina Maxie

Ted had a stroke in 2004, complications from several heart attacks, and diabetes. He became very depressed and developed trouble moving his right hands and legs. Regular doctors gave him the usual course of meds, but it never did any lasting good. Our daughter had heard of Dr. Lucky, so we went to see him. Ted could not travel that far, so the doctor came to us.

He used the Ondamed on him while having him drink water. Suddenly his face got color. I had gone into check on our granddaughter in the pool when 10 minutes later, I was called back to see his stroke-side leg lifting up. He had not done that in a couple of years.

After seeing his blood work, Dr. Lucky adjusted the meds and suggested some vitamins for him to take. It has been a year and a half now; we are unable to go see him because Ted broke his hip, but we still talk to him. Ted is much better now, both emotionally and physically.

While Dr. Lucky was with us, others of his patients came to our home from out of town to see him. I saw one girl diagnosed with Multiple Sclerosis. Dr. Lucky discovered an emotional problem that was causing it. There was another man that came in shaking all over; Dr. Lucky found a problem from his childhood.

Dr. Lucky is not like other doctors. He is smart, intelligent, and has the Lord with him.

The Doctor's Notes:

When Ted came in, he was on a number of medications: ASA, Cozaar, Lasix, Spironolactone, Glucovance, Zieta, Zoloft, Coreg, Lanoxin, Skelaxin. He had four main issues:

1. Four and five vessels CABG's
2. 2004 Heart Failure from Ischemic Cardiomyopathy EF (Ejection Fraction) 10% normal 50-60% and also Left intracerebral hemorrhage with dense hemiparesis (paralysis requiring wheel chair). He had gone to rehab for about 3 years and had seen no further improvement.
3. Left Carotid artery stenosis 100% blocked, 99% Right Carotid Artery Stenosis; underwent Right Carotid endarterectomy in September 2006.
4. Blood sugar issues due to the combination of medications.

I started seeing Ted in August of 2007. At first, he did not want to come see me because it was difficult for him to come over to his daughter's home, which is about two miles away.

Physical Exam: He had a very pale complexion, was in a depressed mood. He had a right carotid artery pulsation normal without bruit and Left no pulse or bruit. Right hand flexion contractures from the stroke laying limp in his lap. Right Foot very purple-black. Right Knee Flexion was almost nothing, and his extension 1-2. (Grades are 5 for full extension against opposition, 4 overcomes gravity, so 1-2 is barely any active movement.)

We discussed emotional issues and did my evaluation to find his issues. That revealed a severe neurovascular component, so we began Ondamed Biofeedback, focusing on the spleen and colon. Spleen indicates an open bleeding wound and colon is an indigestible anger issue. In about 15 minutes, he had a total recovery of his facial complexion, with the largest smile I have ever seen. He began moving his right hand and could actually touch his nose. The most impressive thing that happened, though, was that his right foot turned to normal color after only 45 minutes. He was also able to fully to extend his right knee and his right flexion improved to about 50%. He was able to stand on his own.

Two weeks later, his blood sugar levels began to improve greatly and about one month later, they were dropping into the 50's and 60's.

We also began discontinuing his diuretics because his heart function continued to improve. His kidney function also improved without gaining fluid. He was able to switch to a lower leg ankle brace to strengthen the ankle.

On September 21, his blood sugar continued to run too low, and we began cutting back his Glucovance. He was no longer wearing the ankle brace and we started him on bioidentical testosterone and DHEA, because of some great studies that indicated a reduction of inflammation and improved vascular flow. We were also able to hear bruit on the Left Carotid and reduce upstroke, which indicated the left side was also improving; previously it had been 100% blocked.

The Case Of Kathryn
As Told by Her Mother, Kaycee

Three years ago, my daughter suffered night terrors and was regularly wetting her bed. She also could not use the bathroom without me. The doctors said she would just grow out of all this. Dr. Lucky was recommended to me by a friend, so I decided to try him out.

The first thing he did was scan my daughter's body with his hands, then he asked some questions about my life. I told him how I was hemorrhaging during her delivery, and so she was taken away instead of being given to me, as would be the normal practice. Dr. Lucky's first solution was to pray, then talk with my daughter. She had been afraid of my dying from her first sight of all that blood, and had to check on me in the middle of the night to make sure I was still okay. So, we both had to tell her that I would be okay, that I would never leave her.

He then told us to give her some multivitamins and Vitamin D and sent us home. The night terrors ended.

Dr. Lucky listens very well and I like how he fully explains things. He is always learning and gets excited whenever he learns something new. He listens to new ideas and is not arrogant or proud. Dr. Lucky is enthusiastic, knowledgeable, friendly, and a very good person.

The Doctor's Notes:

While in their town seeing patients, we stayed with our friends for several nights, who have a daughter named Kathryn. Kathryn had been having night terrors; when she needed to use the bathroom, she would arise with a blood-curdling scream, then run to her parent's bedroom and bang on the door until her mother got up and took her to the bathroom. I let this go on for a couple of nights and then I asked the parents what was going on. They told me it was night terrors and that she would grow out of them. I told them she needed to grow out of them tonight, so I sat down with her parents and prayed. Then I scanned her mother's energy; her spleen and bladder showed difficulties. Because of the obvious birth trauma when evaluating for Present time, I asked if she had heavy bleeding with Kathryn's delivery. She said she did. In fact, she had almost died. I then asked her if the nurses had moved Kathryn to another room and she said she believed they did. I told her that Kathryn had a territorial conflict and when she goes to mark her boundaries, she thinks about her mother dying, bleeding to death, and has to check on her in order to go back to sleep. When this was resolved, Kathryn began sleeping through the night with no terrors.

" My people are destroyed for lack of knowledge: because thou hast rejected knowledge, I will also reject thee, that thou shalt be no priest to me: seeing thou hast forgotten the law of thy God, I will also forget thy children. "

Hosea 4:6 KJV Holy Bible

Chapter SEVEN

7 Reasons You Will Die Early & How To Avoid It

There are things going on, both in the world and within yourself that could greatly shorten your life. Fortunately, these things are all easy to avoid once you become aware of them.

1. Not Taking Responsibility

People do not take enough responsibility for themselves or their families. Human nature is to pass the blame, and we see this all around us, from individuals to our government. They would rather pass the blame and make people feel sorry for them. This helps them to feel empowered. We have all been passing the blame since Adam blamed Eve, then Eve blamed the snake. Blame permeates each of our lives, so the key is to start by looking at yourself instead of everyone else. When we do, we will resolve our own problems, and avoid passing them down to our children.

Let us go back to my house metaphor. In this case, there are too many people in the house; they do not have the right priorities, they are very wasteful of their resources, so garbage begins to collect. They are polluting my house. The real issue is not the house, but the people within it. If we will take responsibility for who gets to be in our "house", our bodies will not get to the point where they develop into horrible, chronic, degenerative conditions.

We are the creators of our issues, yet we want to continue to pass the blame. If we will simply accept responsibility for our own problems, even the small things, then things would not get to life-threatening proportions in the first place. By the way, I believe this is even true with the state of our nation. We cannot blame the city or the state governments for the way things are. If we took ownership of our responsibilities, then things would not get to the national level and require such drastic changes.

I have a story that emphasizes this point. About 15 years ago, a young lady came to see me with a history of colon cancer. Her doctors had noticed a mass in her lungs, which they stated, was too close to the vessels to do anything. Because of her age, she elected to do nothing. We placed her on nutrients, performed visualization, and balanced the points that my scan had revealed as abnormal. We found abnormal activity in the L lung corresponding with the X-ray. She also had an imbalance in her L adrenal and splenic areas. We discussed the fear of dying from an open wound.

I then asked her to take the X-ray and pray over it, but when I checked her, I found out that I was going to need to pray over it as well... every day for 30 days. She would then follow up with a CT. Well, after 30 days she refused to have the CT scan. I was disappointed. She finally got the CT and told me they found arthritis in her shoulder, but no mass in her lung. She later displayed a GI bleed with all the symptoms of colon cancer. She said, *"I just knew it."* So I asked why. She said, *"Because the doctor told me it would reoccur."* And she also disclosed that her mother died of the same thing at her age.

When I scanned her, she was much better and my test revealed no abnormal cells, but possibly some diverticula area in the descending colon. I asked her to have a CT scan, which confirmed the known malignancy. We worked on the belief of her "having to have" colon cancer, because the doctor had "told her" it would reoccur. We also addressed the belief that she would not outlive her mother. I explained to her that thoughts were very powerful and could manifest in the tissue. By the way, I learned that day that the reason I was compelled to pray over the x-ray was because I knew that she believed that praying over it was futile.

There are really only two root emotions: love and fear. All we have to do in order to get rid of fear is look in the Bible at 2nd Timothy 1:7 *"For*

God hath not given us the spirit of fear; but of power, and of love, and of a sound mind. There is no fear in love; but perfect love casteth out fear: because fear hath torment. He that feareth is not made perfect in love." Love is the highest frequency there is. It puts you into a sound mind. Fear comes either from the past or from your past interfering with your future. With God, there is only the present! When Moses asked God His name, He said *"I am."*

When we love, we will accept responsibility. We will blame less and live more.

2. Personalization Of Disease

Have you ever said or heard it said, *"My diabetes is out of control."* Or *"my hypertension, my arthritis"* etc.? When we refer to disease this way, we are taking ownership of the disease, which is not too bad initially. You have to realize the problem of owning it, acknowledge it, and then step back a bit. You have to say, *"Ok, what is this? Is this really diabetes? Is it really a disease that is going to progress to dialysis or losing vision? Or is it just blood sugar out of control? And if so, what can I do about these blood sugars to get them under control?"*

If you look at it from that perspective and take control, then you take away the fear of the diagnosis and the dreaded name of the disease and you empower yourself to heal. You need to abandon the disease mindset that owns the label and begin to think in a different pattern, to see things from a different perspective. The question is not *"What can the doctor do for me?"* But rather, *"What can I do for myself?"* I, as your doctor, am merely here to teach you how to remove the obstacles that are between you and perfect health.

So do not look at disease from the perspective of *"Hey, look at me and my diabetes"* but rather *"I think it's time I fixed this. How do I start?"* If you are going to take ownership of anything, try something like *"Hey, look at me. I am young and healthy; that is I. Just a couple of trouble spots, but I can fix those up, then get back to living."*

3. Not Knowing Your Genealogy

Knowing your genealogy is a key to complete health. You would be shocked at the people that do not even know their grandparents or the siblings of their grandparents; or the number of fathers who do not even know the birthdays of their kids. Genealogy linkage allows me to sit down with a patient and help them see how significant their lives are. I also help them see the value of the lives of the loved ones around them. We gain much insight from family connections. Family secrets, for instance, can be very dangerous, so I encourage people to be as transparent as possible about their lives, especially when it comes to their ancestry.

I have seen several histories of traumatic births that the patient did not even know about because someone thought disclosing it might be too hurtful. The problem is that they do not understand that people can die in similar ways. They have similar beliefs and can have events that reappear in their own lives. When I ask about ancestry, I look for a common theme, or a thread that links everything together. Usually I will find a specific linkage pattern with these people and can literally tell how people are going to die, what conditions they will develop, and so on. This allows a very positive shift to occur in their lives.

As mentioned in an earlier chapter, the initial visit begins with a look into the patient's ancestry. In the very least, we go back to their grandparents. I ask about their sibling(s), find out how each person died, what condition they had, and anything else they know about them. It is also key to know about any tragic death events. It helps to know the circumstances surrounding the birth of that person as well as how the pregnancy went. I consider all the pregnancies, including miscarriages, still births, or abortions, because they are a relevant part of the sum total of pregnancies for that person.

This exercise becomes much more difficult for adoptees who may not even know their birth parents. Everyone has a mother and father somewhere, but not knowing more about them can cause a host of disturbances. We are looking at the bloodline, at thought patterns that occur epigenetically, which can begin months prior to conception -- when the parents decide they are ready to have a baby in the first place. The imprint of the beliefs occurs months before the baby's conception. When parents make a decision to have a child, these beliefs begin to download through their ancestry. It is a form of programmed purpose in each of our lives beginning with the birth parents. A direct line of ancestry is very telling, and this is difficult to research with adoptions.

Be careful about deciding on what sex you want your child to be. If you want a boy, but you have a girl, then that child could go through life feeling unwanted, yet not know why. Some prospective parents do not check to see what gender their child is going to be. They just prepare their hearts and the baby room for whatever they want it to be. They decorate in all this beautiful blue because they think it will be a boy, but then it is a girl, so this causes tension and disturbances in the family. This expectation can imprint into the fetus before it is even born. This can cause problems later on if you are not careful.

4. Not Reading Labels

Everyone should know as much as they can about what they put into their bodies. If someone gave you some poison, would you drink it? If someone said that there **might** be poison in something, would you drink it then? What is the cutoff point? Not everything we consume is good for us. This is why reading labels is important.

You see or hear advertisements for a product on radio, television, online, or in the newspaper and blindly trust their advice. There could be cyanide in it, but if it looks tasty enough people will buy it. People are typically much more hesitant to trust products that are not mainstream. If it is a mainstream item that science says could be bad, they are still willing to consume it because it's mainstream. People follow the crowd, even if the product is harmful. They have "psychological glaucoma." The sheep can only see what is in front of their eyes.

My general rule on labels is that if there is anything in there that you do not understand or cannot pronounce, then it is probably not good for you. Start with the first substance listed. This is the most plentiful one in the product, so it has the highest potential effect on you. You also need to look at the inactive ingredients because they actually are not inactive at all. They can have a high negative spin and that is not good for your body.

The fork and spoon can be great instruments of assisted suicide. Whenever we choose 'pleasing the senses' at the expense of the quality of our food, we're in trouble. Low calorie sweeteners, for instance, may not have any calories, but they lead to many other problems. Close to a thousand times stronger than sugar, it causes the body to go into a state of craving more calories to balance out its insulin levels, which compels you to eat more empty calories, and the cycle perpetuates. These food scientists do not place substances in our food to help the body stay healthy. In fact, they are not even necessary for proper function. They are there purely for taste. If you really want to cut down on calories, then eat less food and avoid sugar. If you need to increase your energy, then your mind can help you do that. It can create all the chemicals you need in order to enjoy a satisfying meal, without all the additives.

Aspartame, Splenda, saccharin, and the other artificial sweeteners have the same effect. I have had patients with diabetes who I could never get off their medications until they first got off the artificial sweeteners. They are extremely toxic and increase blood sugar and hemoglobin A1c. Read labels, especially in places you would not suspect: all chewing gums, toothpaste, and medicines; be aware that Sucralose is another name for these artificial sweeteners: Splenda, neotame, aspartame, saccharin, and acesulfame K. Some research show such sweeteners increase obesity and even cause strokes. In general, the more natural, the better. If you must sweeten, then sugar is the better of two possible evils. If you use sugar, avoid refined sugars. You can get enough sugar in fruit, which fiber and enzymes balances blood sugar irregularities.

A 50-year young woman came in with a swollen right knee and had recently had her last allowable steroid shot. They told her she needed surgery very soon. I evaluated her and found toxicity and asked her if she used Splenda. She said she used it every day in her coffee. I told her to stop it immediately. The knee issue resolved the next day. She is currently in her 10th year without any more knee issues.

High fructose corn syrup is another thing to avoid. The manufacturers are aware of its unhealthy effects, so in the future they are going to change the label to read "sugar", so watch out for that. Corn syrup does not cause an insulin surge. Therefore, the body does not know it is full. In addition, it interferes with the hormone ghrelin, which also tells the body it is full, so as a result, you just keep on craving more and more.

MSG (monosodium glutamate) is another dangerous ingredient, one that is very close to my heart...and my stomach...and my eyes. About 15 years ago, I travelled to see a patient. While in town, I stopped by a restaurant that advertises to be healthy. I got a seafood and crab sandwich and about 10 minutes after we left the restaurant, as we were driving down the highway, my left visual field began to develop fan shaped activities. I pulled off the road and let my wife drive the rest of the way. My condition rapidly deteriorated as I lost my sight for about 20 minutes. Then my heart began to race and I became nauseated almost to the point of vomiting.

MSG is an excitatory neuro-stimulant that produces free glutamate and increases insulin levels, most likely damaging part of the hypothalamus, which tells your body when you are full. When MSG hinders this process from fully functioning, one continues to eat. The hypothalamus is also very rich in glutamate receptors that regulate our flight or fight response. MSG and hidden sources of MSG affect people in different ways. You find MSG mostly in processed foods, packaged foods, Chinese food, and Mexican food as a taste enhancer.

Since the time of Adam and Eve, our taste buds have stimulated us. Here is my general rule for grocery shopping. Unless you need healthy spices or a birthday card, shop the outer circumference of the store to obtain fresh and healthier produce. They keep the MSG products on the other shelves.

MSG affects three key areas, which are very rich in glutamate receptors: 1. Heart 2. Gastrointestinal system and 3. Brain. These three systems are there for survival and protection. In nature, food contains some glutamate, but it is the right amount! Too much MSG is associated with cardiac arrhythmia, seizures, nausea, and vomiting. It is not something our bodies require. The addition of MSG is purely to please the pallet, and whatever pleases, sells. It is all about profit, not health.

Have you heard the latest plan to address the problem of obesity? Just change the taste buds! I saw an article asking the question *"Obesity, Are our taste buds the cause?"* The article's author found a random study that claims we have fat sensitive taste buds. Therefore, we need to synthesize new delicious food with less fat or make drugs that block the receptors. What ridiculous nonsense! I want to say, *"Quit messing around with my fat!"*

Do they not know that a function of the taste buds is to protect us from dangerous substances? For example, initially, people do not like artificial sweeteners, but the doctor tells them to use these products because they will be a good substitute for sugar and that there is no harm in consuming them. But the fact is that when you put them in your mouth, they have a bitter taste, which indicates the substance could be poisonous. The researchers' solution to the problem of bitter tasting sweeteners was to harness the chemical that specifically blocks people's ability to detect the bitter aftertaste. Their seemingly wonderful discovery is a molecule known only as GIV3727. According to a report published online in Current Biology, this molecule specifically targets and inhibits a handful of human bitter taste receptors.

Okay so what is the problem? Nobody likes bitter. The problem is that the buds detect the bad! Maybe the people should remind the researchers these bitter taste receptors are there for toxin detection, to keep us safe and alive. On the other hand, maybe they will fall victim to their own "cure" and prove that natural selection works after all! The fact is that God knew what He was doing when He designed our taste buds! Manufacturers, remove the poisons out of our food and quit abusing the bodies of your customers!

I recommend about 80% of your food be in the raw form, or as close to raw as possible; the rest can be broiled or baked. For vegetables, the greener it is, the more vibrant colors, the better it is and the more antioxidants it possesses

Meat is a big problem. It is toxic and putrefied and people eat way too much of it. My rule: if a day's helping does not fit in the palm of your hand, then it is excessively much.

Stay away from Transfats. They increase LDL (the bad cholesterol) and mess up cell membranes. By messing with the cellular membranes, absorption and protection of the cell, you can become more prone to viral infections, allergies, and compromised cellular efficiency needed for energy and electrolytes. The cell membranes are made of a lipid bilayer that is comprised of a mixture of saturated and unsaturated fats. Saturated fats allow the membrane to be stiffer and unsaturated fats allow for kinks and more liquid. Fun fact: That is why butter (a saturated fat) is solid and cold-pressed olive oil (an unsaturated fat) is liquid.

Canola oil is also not good. Not only is it genetically modified, but also when the person heats to high temperature, it causes a trans-configuration that then allows faulty membranes to occur. So stay away from margarine, soy products, and corn oil. Instead, use butter from grass fed cows. Not only is it good for you, but it contains the fat burning agent, activator x, as well as CLA conjugated line oleic acid which help support the immune system, endocrine system, and cardiovascular system. If you do not have access to farm-raised, green pasture, cow butter, then I recommend extra virgin, cold-pressed olive oil or coconut oil (which contains healthy medium chain fatty acids). Another butter benefit is lecithin, which helps with cholesterol deposition. Cholesterol itself is actually a great antioxidant. Cholesterol is very misunderstood in our society. We need to stop this inane fight against cholesterol. Cholesterol is essential for life!

Allergies are never a problem in my clinic. There are many things you can do to get rid of them, and all of them amount to simply taking good care of yourself. In the past, I had severe allergies, along with asthma, that would keep me up all night long. This lasted until I changed my diet about 20 years ago and eliminated transfats. I was extremely allergic to pollen. Earlier, I discussed going outside and getting pollen off my car to imprint homeopathically. I used my finger and had absolutely no issues. Prior to removing trans-fats, I would have had to go to the ER. Most often, simply balancing your body will take care of the allergy.

At all costs, avoid processed food. If you can pick it up at a drive thru window, do not eat it. It is simply not worth your health.

Do not eat pork. It is one of the most unsanitary foods in the world. Think about it; you're eating the meat of an animal who eats slop, has no sweat glands, and whose favorite activity is to roll around in the mud all day.

Read those labels and stay away from transfat oils. Extra virgin olive oil and coconut oil are examples of good oil. But canola oil and anything hydrogenated is just "trans-fat" marketed under a different name.

5. Trusting The Broken Medical System To Fix Us

The fifth thing to avoid that will greatly shorten your life is trusting in the broken medical system. In general, it is not financially solvent and whatever money is left will run out soon. The Government states Medicare and social security are drying up. Each of us must take responsibility for our own health because you cannot trust the system anymore. The system is broken and they are feverishly trying to cut back on expenses, which means cutting back on what they provide for the patient. You have a choice. Will you succumb and say, *"I'm just going to believe what I am being told."* Or will you take a stand and say *"I'm going to test things out and be educated about things and become involved in my healthcare."*

The problem is akin to alcoholism. If you give an alcoholic a drink, he is going to come back for more. People are medical alcoholics, so if you keep on providing the same stuff, they will keep on coming back for more. The way to strengthen the medical system is to straighten yourself out. When you do, you are inhibiting the market that causes all these exorbitant healthcare costs. You will not need all the surgeries they order. You will avoid chronic conditions, and will not be spending most of your money during the last two weeks of your life. Instead, you could use that money to go to Bermuda.

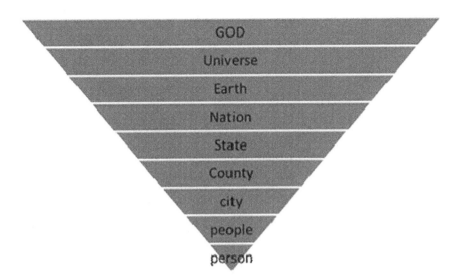

Take care of yourselves, avoid the toxic substances sold in the name of "health", and the broken system might eventually fix itself. Learn how to love people, love the Lord with all your heart, soul, mind, and strength, and love your neighbor. If we do these things, we will not have the problems that we do in the world today. We created every single one of these problems. We are the ones that broke the system.

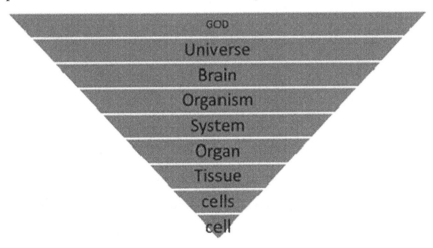

There are two health care programs working today. One kills and the other gives life. This sounds very much like a verse in the bible.

1. The thief cometh not but to steal, kill and destroy.

2. I come to give you life and life more abundantly.

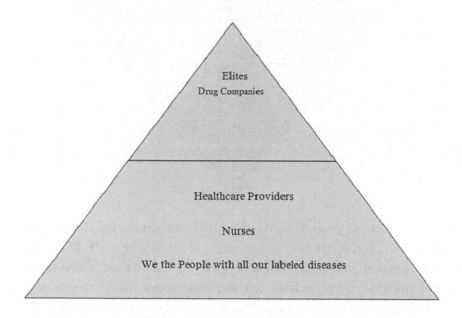

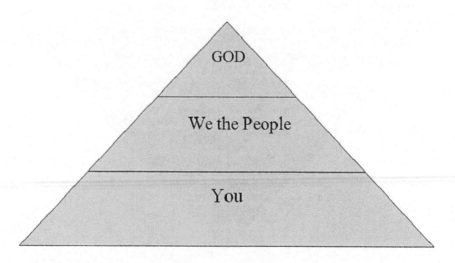

We have to put God back on the throne of our lives where He belongs!

Satan's Plan is a plan of lack! God's Plan is a plan of abundance!

Features of Satan's plan:

Alter the food and the body from natural use that brings no value except to the industry and weakens society.

Change herbs that had been safe for thousands of years to make drugs that are toxic and patentable.

God's simple plan:

Change people's hearts and lives to the betterment of society.

Help mankind realize how much God values him.

Keep it simple. God is into simplicity not complexity.

One has to realize how big God is relative to how small your problems is. In Mississippi, around late March or early April, we have the flowering of the Pear Blossom tree. It is always there, but only when it blossoms does it stand out from all the other trees. As human beings, we do not notice things or people until something happens that gets our attention, even though it or they have been there all along. You go to the doctor and even though you have had symptoms for a while, you have ignored them or denied them as being serious. But when the doctor tells you that you have "X" disease, it gets your attention. You begin focusing on the diagnosis, you spend hours googling as you investigate your options, researching into the wee hours of the night, asking questions of friends and family members and getting their opinions. What your fearful reaction solidifies is a level of panic that is much more destructive than the disease process. Our focus is in not on God and His power, but on the disease and its power over us.

God has never left the scene and He is much larger than any of our problems. But apparently we believe this diagnosis happened over night and only conventional medicine can help us by either burning, poisoning, or cutting it out. The media programs us to think this way, so we conform. Medical doctors only deal with the physical, which is the root problem about ten percent of the time. Even the Center for Disease Control states that 80% of our health issues are rooted in emotions, but even psychiatric medicine is not the answer.

The bible states in Psalm 23: *"The Lord is my shepherd... and He maketh me to lie down in green pastures."* When you lie down, it causes you to rest and grow. When you do not rest your body and brain, bad things happen and those bad things grow. When we rest and relax, we experience, we hear, we feel, and we see with our heart things that have always been there, but we were too busy to recognize them; or we ignored or denied them.

In August of 2015, I became ill with sudden onset of severe gastroesophageal reflux issues, released about 20 pounds, and had left abdominal pain and extreme fatigue. It felt like a knife was stabbing me in my back and exiting through my chest. Two trusted friends told me that I was dying and needed to plan my funeral. Prior to getting ill, I had totally compromised my health by taking on a very demanding schedule at the clinic for a solid week. I was not eating, nor was I drinking enough water. I was working with seriously ill people, from eight am until ten pm each day. I was not seeing my family and I felt manipulated by the people I was attempting to help. A root of bitterness consumed me and it was quite destructive to my family life.

One of my wonderful clients suggested I go to Georgia to a holistic clinic for a week. Instead, I went on a 2,000 mile round trip to a clinic in Florida and wasted a month of precious time. This was after I had tried everything from supplements to relaxation therapies, from guided imagery to autosuggestions, from chiropractic to MD's. And no, I did not use prescription medicines. I used every device in my clinic, but had minimal improvement.

I became quite discouraged and had to get away from all emails, text messages, Facebook communication and especially the clinic. I began to journal about all the events I knew in my life and some things I did not even know about. Then a wonderful client family told me they wanted me to go to Wildwood for a week. I agreed.

At Wildwood, I really benefited from being able to rest and walk in the mountains by myself. Then one day while I was walking and complaining to God about my situation, it was as if a light from heaven came down and stopped me in my tracks. God showed me that I had traded my Isaac for Ishmael. In Genesis, God promised elderly Abraham a son, but he jumped ahead of God's promise and produced a son named Ishmael, rather than waiting for God to produce Isaac. God had given me a promise, but I had also chosen second best. I took the provision of the flesh over what God had promised me. I cried out to the Lord, *"Give me my Isaac back and things will be different."*

The next day, I went to do my hydrotherapy treatment and would you not know it, my therapist's name was Isaac! Don't tell me that God doesn't have a sense of humor! At Wildwood, each procedure I went through the staff preceded and completed with prayer. God was there!

What I am saying in all of this is that I had to get my focus back on Jesus and get my focus off my problem. I had been dwelling on the wrong things. When I allowed myself to get to a place where I could rest my body and brain, I was once again able to hear, feel, and experience what my heart needed, and my body healed.

The place I went to in Florida had recommended that I give the middle finger to my wonderful, 91-year young father and curse him out for programming me with a poverty mindset. That was an Ishmael mindset, completely contrary to the heart of God. There was, however, one good thing that came out of my time in that clinic…I learned to use wheat grass every way you could possibly imagine!

Take care of yourself. Avoid the toxic substances sold in the name of "health." Learn how to love people. Love The Lord your God with all your heart, soul, mind, and strength. Love your neighbor. When we all do these things, we will not have the problems that we have in the world today.

6. No Commitment

Another dangerous toxin is our unwillingness to commit. This causes people to experience failure in life. In previous generations, a handshake was a person's bond. Today, going to a lawyer is a person's bond. Why? Because we do not trust each other.

A cow participates in your breakfast by providing the milk, but the pig **commits** to your breakfast by giving its life. That is the difference between participating and committing. Most people participate. Doctors participate. We all participate in the health care system, but too few actually commit to good health. You have to learn how to commit to your health. Talk is cheap, but actions bring results.

You need to commit to at least 3 months. About 80-90% of people will improve within the first month. Some of them improve almost instantaneously in our clinic. If they are not better within a month, then it is usually because they are not doing what I told them to do. I have ways of finding out if they are doing what they are supposed to be doing. They usually 'fess up by the end of our two-hour appointment, at which point I tell them *"That's why you're not doing well yet."* They are wasting their time and money.

You must be committed to exercise and doing the things that I have being saying throughout this book:

Be faithful with the visualization exercises.

Be faithful with the breathing exercises.

Be faithful to eat the super green foods, especially things like wheat grass juice, chlorella, and spirulina.

Be faithful to the quality of the foods in your diet.

If you can be committed for the first three months, then you have the rhythm. You will then understand what it takes. You will be better off and your body will thank you for it and reward you handsomely.

7. Believing the Lie

"It's just too expensive to be healthy!" Most people believe this lie, but actually, the opposite is true. Take care of your health and your health will take care of you. Then when you are healthy, you will not need to make the expensive hospital visits that break your budget.

Some people believe that the Bible teaches that we are only supposed to live until about 70 or 80 years of age. If we live longer, they believe that we must be doing something unnatural. That is another popular lie. The Bible does tell of how people back in that day would live until about 70 or 80, but nowhere does it say, "Thou shalt not live past 80 years of age." When people get to a certain age, they expect that bodily degeneration is perfectly normal, so they accept it and allow it to happen, instead of taking the same care for themselves as they did when they were younger.

If you believe a thing, you can make it true. Believe in a lie and the lie becomes the reality; believe in something positive and that will happen instead. I have had many cases in which a patient's belief was the causative factor in both their illness and in their miraculous recovery. So the next time someone tells you that whatever positive and hopeful thing you are going for is "impossible" or "unrealistic," just nod politely and ignore them. Refuse the lie.

The Case Of KT from Michigan

I would come down to see my aunt, who had onset Alzheimer's, when I decided to seek Dr. Lucky for his help. I would cough before bed, sometimes coughing up blood, had no stamina, could not walk or work for very long, and I had night sweats. This went on for months. Doctors said I had an infection. My family physician said I had a severe heart murmur, 4 on scale of 1 to 5. Ultrasound showed a faulty valve, with blood going back into my lungs to cause the cough, and an angiogram showed clogged veins and a need for a by-pass and valve surgery. I had been on medications for the heart and blood pressure, but had stopped after 1 year because I could not tolerate the side effects.

Dr. Lucky put me on supplements, used the Ondamed, muscle treatments, other treatments, and prayed for me. After 4 to 5 months, the coughing was reduced. Before, simply walking up or down hill would be difficult, but now I can walk and even use a bucksaw again.

Dr. Lucky has a strong integrity, is very spiritual, of good cheer, and very peaceable. He is quite an unusual doctor.

The Doctor's Notes:

Patient states he was having cough and actually coughing up blood at times, night sweats for several months. Patient stated that when he lies down to bed he coughs about half an hour before going to sleep. On 12/09/2005, I recommended CXR and that he needed to go to the clinic. He was concerned about his hormones and the role they may be playing. He went to the hospital and the Physician's Assistant did not have enough experience to read the X-ray, but he felt a little enlarged spleen and believed the sinus drainage caused the blood-tinged sputum. The doctor treated him with Doxycycline and cough medication.

A previous X-ray showed a shadow and I wanted to know what the comparison X-ray showed. I also explained something bad could be going on, and before just treating with antibiotics, I wanted to know about the shadow.

Patient stated he could walk effortlessly before as far as he wanted, but now half a block was taxing.

Patient saw his doctor on December 19 and he found a questionable aortic murmur that was large, and the EKG tracing went off the sheet. I told him this was serious and needed immediate attention. The doctor ordered an ECHO which was performed a couple days later, indicating moderate, enlarged Left atrium and severe mitral regurgitation and chordal rupture on posterior leaflet. The heart maintained LV systolic function but the severe mitral regurgitation exaggerated the findings. The reversal was back flowing into the pulmonary veins. He also had severe tricuspid regurgitation and an increased pulmonary pressure of 60-65. They wanted him to do surgery immediately.

He was placed on Coreg and Avapro, but could not have surgery because his VA benefits were not in order. In the meantime, he asked me to help him balance his nutritional state. He had already begun Cardio plus and some other vitamins.

The patient told me via email that he had reduced activity and was therefore "doing ok." I saw him on January 14 of 2006 and upon evaluation, he was very frail with a BP of 105/68, PR of 65 CV sitting in the chair, jugular venous distention (JVD) to the angle of the jaw, and obvious shortness of breath. When he talked much, he would begin to cough in spasms. RRR with 6/6 mitral regurgitation with radiation into the L axilla. Lungs had some bibasilar crackles or rales.

I evaluated him energetically and found he had a severe heart issue with the mitral valve area very weak along with adrenal weakness, thyroid weakness, and spleen. We discussed counter clockwise maneuvers to try to strengthen the valve and placed him on nutrition including the glyconutrients at very high amounts, and prayed.

On January 26, 2006, I received an email from KT: *"Shoveled some snow yesterday that I wouldn't have been able to do a month ago. Walked to the store and back ok this afternoon, about half mile where previously I would have had to stop twice. "*

About a year later, he stopped all the prescription meds and continued to do well hiking up a 3200 foot pathway that included long, 60 degree grades of steps without difficulty.

The Case Of Charlene Shortridge
As Told by Reverand Allen Shortridge

On June 12, 2001, my first wife Charlene Shortridge was at a church service and had a violent seizure. The emergency techs took her to the ER where she regained consciousness. They did some CAT scans and found a large mass on the right front portion of her brain. They then urged me to take her to a university hospital, but I held off. That was on a Tuesday. The following Friday I took her to Dr. Lucky.

He examined her and her CAT scan. He then sent her to the ER at the University Medical Center in Jackson and did a MRI, biopsy, and found it was a type of fast acting tumor.

On June 19, she had surgery to reduce the tumor. She was then told that she had 6 months left to live, perhaps more with aggressive chemo therapy. We said no to the chemo, which angered the doctors. We stuck with Dr. Lucky and for 16 months things were okay.

In November of 2002, she had another seizure and it was back to the ER; the tumor had returned. Back to Dr. Lucky and he put her on natural supplements, then I put her in the hospice. The hospice nurse said she had 2 weeks to live, but she pulled through and continued to drive and walk as a normal person. Dr. Lucky continued to visit her in both the hospice and in our home. By June 4, 2003, she had one more seizure, but a brain scan revealed that the tumor had shrunk to the size of a small nut. She had no problems until March of 2004 when she had another seizure. We continued treatments and hospice, but after so much time in hospice, they send you to a nursing home. The nursing home would not allow us to give her the supplements that Dr. Lucky recommended and so on January 27, 2007 she finally died. The doctors said it was amazing that she had survived the initial seizure, much less lived that long, especially with no chemo or radiation treatment.

Dr. Lucky uses no drugs, just all supplements and a healthy diet. He also uses prayer, a special light, and some healing herbs from South America. He also *looks into the emotional causes. He helped encourage her when she nearly gave up. Charlene lived 6 times longer than normal for her type of tumor, and was fully aware of everything around her right up until just before she passed away.*

Doctor Lucky is phenomenal and compassionate. His goal is to see people get well.

The Doctor's Notes:

Charlene Shortridge: The Pastor's wife who doctors diagnosed her with Glioblastoma Multiforme in 2001. We sent her to Jackson and they did a craniotomy with removal of most of the tumor. Then we placed her on a few nutrients, but the tumor came roaring back and in Nov 2002, so she went to the ER with seizures; CT Brain scan revealed a huge frontal lobe tumor with blood and significant fluid deviating the midline of the brain due to the excessive pressure. The doctor placed her on home hospice and pain medication, anxiety meds, seizure meds, steroids. She allowed me to be her doctor and we made many trips to her home.

Her husband had to lift her by himself from the extreme weakness on her right side, but within two weeks, she began to walk on her own. We had previously discontinued her pain and anxiety medications, but left her on a reduced amount of steroids and seizure medications. Her facial weakness and slurred speech resolved. We prayed frequently, placed her on glyconutrients, juicing, melatonin, and antioxidant support and she continued to improve enough to drive her car and play the piano. After about three months, in February, a repeat scan indicated no blood, no obvious mass, and the midline deviation resolved. We took her off steroid medications and tapered off the seizure medications.

She did well and had no issues, but about 18 months later, she had another bad seizure and taken to the hospital. This time the ambulance took her to a different hospital, but the CT scan actually looked better than the previous CT scan. The hospital discontinued the nutrients and our program, and the tumor quickly returned. The doctor admitted her to the hospital, and she was in great pain, which required pain medication. I did not play as active a role this time because her husband was unable to take care of her at home. The doctors admitted her to inpatient hospice where they controlled her meds, but we were able to get her back on the nutrients so she did improve enough to get her back to walking down the hall with some help.

She stayed in fairly good shape for a combined six years without chemo, radiation, or other medical treatment. When people do not die on hospice, the hospital will discharge the person. Because the concerned husband was not able to take care of her by himself, and she was not deteriorating, In-patient hospice placed her in the nursing home. The nursing home refused to allow the nutritional agents to be used, so she rapidly deteriorated and died several months later.

This case indicates the awesome power of God and how His ways can help a person when the person has determination.

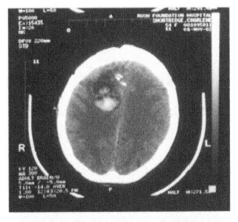

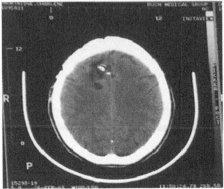

November 1, 2002 -February 26, 2003

" Water is the most neglected nutrient in your diet, but one of the most vital "

-Julia Child

Summary

This book has been about healing, about obtaining and maintaining optimal health and reversing the fiction of the chronological aging process. Healing must be for more than simply the physical body. The brain, heart, and body are integrated; parts of the same whole. Therefore, the state of one can affect the other. A person in a depressed mood, who does not feel he can get better, will not; heart will limit what his body can do. Likewise, some physical conditions can affect the mood of a person. As a result, as Brain, Body, and Spirit are together as a whole, then we must treat as a whole. That is the principle of my practice and my personal beliefs.

From there, I have developed a program that **helps the body to heal itself**, for God created the body to heal that way. I focus on healthy diet and supplements, detoxing the body, and keeping body and mind fit and young. From those simple precepts seeming miracles can occur. All I do as a physician is listen to the patients, listen to their bodies, and empower them to heal themselves.

Seven Simple Principles summarizes full and permanent healing. Follow these principles and you too can perform miracles upon your body. In addition, remember, God performs healing only in the Present. What happened in the Past or might happen in the Future do not determine your healing.

1) **Heart:** Take responsibility for your health, be a victor instead of a victim. You cannot heal if you do not commit to it.

2) **Thought Blocks Health:** What you think, your beliefs and hidden emotional issues can be preventing your body from healing. Recognize and deal with these issues and the healing will commence.

3) **Release the Negative Power:** Wrong or mistaken beliefs can cause disease. By severing the beliefs that are hindering you, you cut off the disease's power over you.

4) **Fuel Your Body Right:** Your body needs the proper nutritional support, the right raw materials with which to rebuild and maintain itself.

5) **Fueling Your Brain:** It is just as important to exercise your Brain as it is your Body. Get out of the rut of linear thinking and expand your mental capabilities.

6) **Rapid Healing:** Once the heart is balanced, the Body and Brain in synch, then healing begins immediately.

7) **The #1 Healing Mechanism Is The Heart:** The heart is what it's all about. The body follows its commands, so only when the heart sends the correct message to the brain that the body can get better will true healing occur. Miracles of healing have occurred simply through the proper belief.

My last piece of advice is to follow through. Reinforce yourself with new beliefs, new nutrition, and new exercises. Maintain an awareness of what your body and heart need and keep an open mind to the fact that there are more things in Heaven and Earth than are dreamt of in the annals of mainstream medical practice.

Many people have told me they do not have the funds for our treatment, but they do have the desire. I have to compromise my time and money because I cannot let these people die over money if they have a desire to live. In the future, I dream and envision a charity arm of the clinic where people who lack funds but have a desire to be well can come. My greatest motto in life is always to do what is right and not always popular. I have to have a clean conscience that I did all that I could do to help my fellow friend. Many times, people I have seen have given up, and I do not want to have to answer to God. The charity will not enable people but teach how people can be well and be good stewards of their health and wealth so they can help others. Every three months each person would have an evaluation according to need and their compliance to their health program, and if they are not in compliance, the release process will commence.

My other dream is to have a holistic treatment facility that allows people to spend about 3 days for aggressive evaluation, organic healthy eating, and learning how to live a totally holistic life and teach others also. My motto in life is we all need a teacher until we learn we are the teacher and can now teach others.

" Now faith is the substance of things hoped for, the evidence of things not seen. "

Hebrews 11:1 KJV Holy Bible

Chapter EIGHT

The Faith Chapter

———————◄◆►———————

The number 8 in the Greek is theta and the number 8 on its side is the infinity sign. The frequency for our white blood cells, and thus immune system is 8 cycle/sec. The principles of the word of God are based on the number 8. I feel that God has given us a chapter 8 as a bonus that will definitely help your brain, heart, and body to heal.

The way the body works is like a computer system, albeit the most sophisticated computer system in the universe. The information comes in through the senses, which integrates in the brain, then searches the heart for memories in the catalog of life. If the brain is the CPU, the heart is the Hard Drive, our belief systems are the Operating System on the hard drive, and our thoughts are the programs running on and utilizing the operating system. But just as a computer can acquire a virus that compromises its functionality, our thoughts can become infected with a virus (negative thoughts) and spread among the programs we are running in life. If it is not recognized and caught, it can spread throughout our network (the people around us) and cause quite a bit of damage. Our thoughts imprint onto our hearts to protect us from danger using multi-dimensional images (vibrations). Our thoughts have to travel through our belief systems, and if our belief systems are not congruent with our thoughts, it creates the emotion of fear in order to protect us. It sees fear as an image, involving all the senses of sight, sound, smell, tactile stimulation, and taste. It then connects it with the event that is happening, searching for a similar day, time, event or image and retrieves it to resolve the past issue. Virtual reality is as powerful as reality. See a rubber snake that looks real and some people would react with terror. Your body does not appear to know the difference.

There are only two basic emotions from which all others emanate, Love and Fear. In the Garden of Eden, we saw this illustrated when Adam and Eve hid themselves from God out of Fear. They then proceeded with Anger, Guilt, and Shame. The devil (as the serpent) asked the question *"Yea, hath God said, ye shall not eat of every tree of the Garden?"* The Serpent was asking the question out of lack not out of abundance. His question got Eve to focus on the limitations instead of the abundance that God had for them. Void is what drives a person, not Abundance. There are three basic fears: (1) Being Bored (2) Of becoming nothing (3) Ceasing to exist. All our fears end with these conditions if we continue to think deeper.

Adam said, *"The woman whom thou gavest to be with me, she gave me of the tree and I did eat."* We project our issues onto our loved ones instead of taking responsibility ourselves. God places a mirror in front of us every day so we can better learn who we are. But we focus on the other people, and how they done us wrong, instead of how we have failed and need to learn from that situation. Adam did not have to eat that fruit, but he did and should have accepted 100% of the responsibility. He felt guilty and projected it onto Eve.

We have to take into captivity every thought! We should examine our thoughts to determine whether the thought is serving us in a positive manner. Paul stated in Philippians 4:8, *"Finally, brethren, whatsoever things are true, whatsoever things are honest, whatsoever things are just, whatsoever things are pure, whatsoever things are lovely, whatsoever things are of good report; if there be any virtue, and if there be in praise, think on these things."* If only we would have thoughts like these, our belief systems would not be so toxic to us.

We have the formation of our belief systems early in development. We look at our parents as our God figures. They brought us into this world and taught us to conform, so they are the primary influence on how we define love for the rest of our lives. If they verbally or physical abuse one another or us, we begin to think this is a representation of what love is, so we look for a match in the people around us.

Our nation is full of people like you and me who need healing of the misrepresentations of love. One place to start is to guard your eyes. I believe that if God is going to heal the nation, we need to eliminate the sewage pipe that comes into our homes from Hollywood. We also need to remove the video games that promote violence. As parents, we should be very careful to monitor what we allow in our homes. The images from computers and televisions imprint holographically into our children's hearts, and they become like what they see and hear. This is why kids are killing kids in schools. Folks, it is not rocket science!

You must remember that the body is mainly water and light and everything is imprinting on it; toxic words lead to toxic chemicals.

The Holy Bible says, *"To love the Lord with all your heart, soul, mind, and strength."* and *"to love your neighbor as yourself."* Your closest neighbor is yourself. You must learn to love yourself before you can really love anyone else. It is like a ripple effect. You throw a rock into the water, and from the center, the ripple spreads out. You are the rock, and your perception of life affects everything in the universe. The problem is that people do not really love themselves. They hate themselves. At their heart level, the average person feels unworthy, undesirable, rejected, and undeserving.

Remember it took one sperm cell (out of 100,000,000!) and one egg to get you here on this planet called earth. 99,999,999 cells had to die (sacrifice) in order for you to get here! No two people are alike. Just look at the uniqueness of fingerprints. Yet in the middle of this miracle of originality, there is a global movement to make us all the same.

You have a purpose. Your life has meaning. There is a specific reason that God has put you on earth at this moment in time. Find your passion and your potential is unlimited. You are not a "piece of junk." You are precious in the sight of God. Do not limit yourself. You have a purpose that is greater than yourself.

Your thoughts, positive or negative, go through the filters of your beliefs and produce emotions. You must obtain trust in your beliefs, but to gain trust, you must have knowledge. The reason people do not get well is that they only intellectually believe they can get well. It is much deeper than that! They must trust in what they believe and take responsibility and accountability, without the need to blame someone else.

When you love someone, you want to know all about that person so that you can trust him or her. Similarly, knowledge is what gives you power for the healing to take place. Faith is unshakable when you know that healing will occur. However, how do you counter your unbelief? Build knowledge on both sides of the equation: conventional vs. natural healing methods. Then make decisions based on what you discover. When someone comes to see me who is terminal, as far as the medical establishment is concerned, I always have them ask their body this question just prior to going to sleep: *"Why is my body doing what it is doing?"* Then, the next time I see them, I have them ask, *"Why are my cells so healthy and working harmoniously together for the good of my body?"* You have to empower the seesaw of thoughts in your favor, not according to someone else's belief systems.

The accepted medical standard of care is a way to globalize everything into slots, which consists of labels. The goal is for you to own that label. Possession is powerful and it can become your identity. The advertisers have 15, 30 or 60 seconds on television to promote fear in a person that is experiencing nothing more than the normal symptoms from simply not taking care or eating like he should. They give him a solution that is actually worse than the symptoms themselves, then at the end of the commercial they ask the question: *"What are you going to do about your _____?"* They are in the business of contracting you with an illness so you will go get a diagnosis (label) out of fear, then put you in a contract with the pharmaceutical company so you will be a client for life. You will pay the doctor (the contract establishing value with a hopeless situation) and then you will pay the pharmacist (another contract).

The doctor is only looking at the body as a mechanical instrument, so he intends to treat you by blocking or stimulating a physiological process that has gone awry. The Holy Bible says, *"Whatsoever you bind on Earth will be bound in Heaven and whatsoever you loose on Earth will be loosed in Heaven."* You come into agreement (bind through contracting) so that is why you keep your label and your so called disease that someone has manufactured for you. You are now in bondage to something that is only powerful in the eyes of man and actually has no power. You make it powerful when you decide to own it!

Adam named all the animals because God gave him dominion over them. You have taken on a name associated to nothing but hopeless symptom management. This action pushes the problem deeper, and there is no solution except drugs, surgery, radiation, and/or chemotherapy. You have conformed to the label, yet you wonder why you are sick! You are essentially under a spell and you do not even know it! This is not building faith. It is building fear!

One major obstacle to faith is our families. They do not mean to cause a problem, and usually they really want to help, but many times, they harm more than help. They have guilt programs that they should not have when one of their loved ones become terminally ill. They want the person to live, when much of the time the person just wants permission to go on and have their reward in heaven. Out of fear, they start using every kind of potion—cream, vitamin supplement, oil, and device they can find to try to help. Sometimes you have to treat the family instead of the client that originated the visit.

Another obstacle to faith is the healthcare provider. Sometimes, a patient visits a physician and he is more panicked than the patient is over the condition. The patient needs to tell the physician *"It's going to be okay."* Then check his pulse to make sure he actually is okay! Doctors can destroy a person's faith very quickly by telling them that they have a limited amount of time left.

Several years ago, I had a client who had terminal colon cancer and was vomiting and passing blood and was pale as a white sheet. She looked like death personified and I thought she might die in my office. Her husband brought her 300 miles to see me because the oncologist had told her that she was not a candidate for treatment because the cancer had progressed too far. Two weeks after her visit, I called her and she was out mowing the grass and feeling great. She told me she was going to see her oncologist. I asked her why and her husband also tried to convince her not to see him. I told her that the doctor had given up on her, that she was feeling much better, so why would she go back and see someone that could offer her no further options. In spite of our counsel, she went back to see the doctor who said that since she looked so much better, she was strong enough to try chemo. She did and the first round of chemo resulted in her death.

Society conditions us to believe that the doctors are our authority figures and we need to submit to whatever they tell us to do. We unwittingly deify our loving physicians who take care of us from conception to death. I am not suggesting that you should not pay attention to the doctor. I am suggesting that you should listen, and then see if what they are saying is really true.

When our parents conceive, they carry us to the doctor to confirm our mother is pregnant. Throughout the pregnancy, you visit the doctor and the mother conforms to what the doctor says to do. Sometimes the first male voice a child hears is the doctor's. When you are born, your parents run to the hospital as if they need to manage a disease and the doctor brings us into this world and gets a nice paycheck that he or she deserves.

We have many wonderful doctors in the world who sincerely want to help people, but physicians should not belittle their patient's opinions nor make quick judgments about something they know nothing about. You cannot just destroy a person's beliefs. They are foundational. When you increase knowledge and have an open heart, unlimited potential can unfold.

Three words I use every day: "I Don't Know"

The 98% rule:

1. What the doctor knows he knows = 1%
2. What the doctor knows he doesn't know = 1%
3. What the doctor doesn't know that he doesn't know = 98%

Why we "do not know"

1. There are more bacteria in your body than the number of cells and we still do not know their function.
2. There are an estimated 100 trillion cells in your body.
3. Your total circulatory system stretches out estimated 60,000 miles.
4. The liver has over 500 different functions and this is why we call it the LIVEr.
5. The brain has over 100 billion neurons with their different connections.
6. You have about 100 thousand miles of lymph vessels.

With so much complexity, it's fitting that a physician is said to have a medical "practice." Do we as physicians really know what we are doing or are we just practicing?

There is a simple system called fractals that God uses that confounds the knowledge of humanity. Everything in nature is fractals, which are iterations of the same thing. Just cut down a tree and look at the rings or the branches of the tree, and view the nodes on the limb. Observe the distance between the nodes, and if you cut it in two, you would see a similar design. The mAcrocosm looks the same as the mIcrocosm. As it is above, so it is below. Now, look at the human being If you were to cut through the aorta you would find a vessel as large as a garden hose that continues to branch until it is the size of a capillary which is microscopic (one capillary equates to the thickness of ten human hairs). We are fearfully and wonderfully made. John the Baptist stated: *"He must increase, but I must decrease.."* John 3:30 KJV

As physicians, we should be humbled that God's creations trust us with their bodies, the most precious part of their lives. We should not be driven by our egos and look at the patient as someone who is lower on the totem pole, food chain, or pecking order. When the sperm and the egg unite to form the first cell of your body, the cells will continue to divide to form 2,4,8,16,32,64,128,256... ... ...cells, until you become an organism made up of many systems. The most powerful moment in the creation of a child occurs at the one cell level and everything that it needs for life and your entire duration on earth is present in that cell.

If you knew how powerful this is and the way one can harness the free energy from this system and visualize themselves back to health, we would have much less illness today.

So how do you start? You have to humble yourself and value yourself to be healed. You must lose the fear of dying and the need to have to depend on someone else or the need to support someone else. You must take care of yourself first! At our clinic, we want clients who are committed to take control of their lives for the challenge that lay ahead of them. You must erect boundaries where nothing matters but God and you. You must live your day as if it is the last day for you on earth. You must change your perspective and have an about face, because if you do not you will continue toward destruction.

Recently, I developed a headache and it was pretty bad. I never take medicine for the pain, because pain is a good indication I did something wrong and my body needs to rectify it. I was feeling the full effect of the headache! I began focusing on how 99.5% of my body was painless so I focused on that and within 5 minutes the headache was history.

We automatically give more negative energy to what is bothering us instead of the areas that are feeling great. I like to call it my 99 vs. 1 program and it gets its inspiration from the Bible. Jesus left 99 and sought out the 1 lost sheep. Sheep are gentle, timid animals, but when something or somebody harms them, it is very difficult to earn back their trust. Jesus left the 99 and found the 1 that was lost, then placed it near His ear and spoke gently to it, explaining how much He cared for it, and how deeply He loved it.

This is similar to tumor development. Only about 1% of the cells of a tumor are malignant. These cells are primitive stem cells that do not want to die so they devise survival mechanisms to prevent their demise. The more you try to kill them, the more alternative mechanisms they create. I am opposed to war on anything, especially when it comes to the body. I do not like it when doctors use disease-fighting terminology such as killing, fighting, or destroying because there is too much friendly fire going on.

I was discussing this idea and relating it to the war on cancer with a patient who had an abnormal cell history. Her friend, who had accompanied her to the visit, had been seeing an oncologist. As I told her, what needs to happen and how we need to nurture these abnormal infant-like cells and love them back to the fold. The friend grabbed her breast and stated, *"It's gone!"* That concerned me because I thought maybe her breast disappeared, but she had had a tumor and it just disappeared.

Life is a process of learning to strive for perfection, but if we fall along the way, we just need to pull ourselves up and keep going. We might have failed several times in life, but that does not make us a failure. The word "Cancer" has powerful negative connotations. Instead, what if we referred to the problem as "abnormal cell development?" This term carries with it very little negative energy and implies the condition is a process that can reverse itself.

You can easily reverse a "process," but it is more difficult to stop something that is already at its "final stage." Words matter! If you must use the word cancer, it would be better to say something like *"my body is cancering."* Why are we so compelled to refer to anything except the process? Ask the question *"why?"* (reason) and the how (process) will come.

When you call someone's name, he or she is more likely to look than when you call for them by title: father, mother, brother, sister or friend. **The name is where the power is**, so if the doctor has pronounced a disease label, then you have given your identity and power over to that label. Even in the practice of hospital-based medicine, in conversations among the doctors, they refer to patients not by their names, but by their condition: "There's a Gallbladder in Room 5…Myocardial Infarction Room 2…and Room 8 is a seizure." Your disease or organ became your identity. You have to get your personhood back in order to heal because it is your true identity.

The Holy Bible is into numbers and genealogy. There are whole books dedicated to these topics. I like to look at the Holy Bible and at nature for my answers in life. Even if God did not exist, I would still not go wrong by applying the bible's morals, ethics, laws, and health precepts to my life. Among so many other things, it teaches us to live within boundaries. Without boundaries, you can feel as if there is nothing in life. When you feel as though you may become nothing, it incites great fear. Animals have boundaries that they mark. We also need boundaries and we need to respect other people's boundaries.

People generally want control, but what we really need is to understand that only God is in control. Only God knows the big picture and only He sees the end result. One area of control that we hold to with great fervor is reproduction. The word of God is clear that we are to be fruitful and replenish the earth. Therefore, anything that controls birth is not of God and promotes death. (Birth control pills, tubal ligation, vasectomy). When a sperm and egg come together, you get a fertilized cell called a zygote, which continues to grow until it is a full-grown man or woman. Who are we to decide whether God needs his children on the earth? Birth control pills are also bad for your health. They are associated with blood clots, malignancy, migraines, yeast infections, autoimmune disease, etc.

We do not control much of anything that is important. Instead of taking responsibility to raise our precious children, we allow Hollywood to babysit them, teaching them its perverted version of right and wrong. We simply do not have time to be with them, most often due to our busyness. The TV becomes their authority figure instead of their parents. God gives children to the parents and they are not the responsibility of the village or global community. WE need to get back to the basics of our calling by bowing down on our knees, humbling ourselves, turning from our wicked ways, and seeking the face of God.

I saw a gentleman several years ago who came to me with severe edema. He had developed severe cirrhosis of the liver from fatty liver and required abdominal paracentesis with replacement of albumin every two weeks. His last tap was 6 weeks prior to our initial visit and he was taking spironolactone, Lasix, and other meds. His diet was not good. His MELD score was 12, which indicates the severity of the end stage liver condition. We discussed boundaries. We pointed to an event from 1979 when he was driving a blue truck at about 25 mph when a lady ran a stop sign. In the cab of the truck with him were two men, one of whom was blind. One of the friends had some dogs in the back of the truck. Following the accident, his father had shamed him for not watching more carefully. We discussed forgiveness and not having the need to sacrifice for anyone as well as the need to establish boundaries for himself. Since our meeting, he has never had to see me again and never had any more collection of fluid requiring paracentesis.

A gentleman in his 60's came to me diagnosed with hepatocellular carcinoma by three of the most prestigious cancer centers in America. He was comatose and having severe asterexis from liver failure, which required removal of 25 pounds of fluid from his abdomen every 2 weeks. He was in kidney failure with BUN 125 and a creatinine of 10, but could not have a transplant because of the 8 cm mass in his liver. His family nearly dragged him in by wheelchair and his skin was very yellow in color. He had not urinated in the past week. His desire was to be able to get a liver and kidney transplant.

We did what we do in the clinic, but when he returned home, his family believed that he should not have come because his eyes were all sunken in and rolled back. I told him he could just be resetting and might wake up the next day a different person or he could be dying. They called in the family minister to give him his last rites, but on that same day, he happened to get out of bed, stood up behind his wheelchair and pushed it into the room! Also on that day, he began urinating and getting rid of all the excess fluid. Three days after that, he was walking in the mall!

Sadly, he never returned to me, but rather went to see all the other doctors who stated that he was dying and that there was nothing else to do but hospice. He lived about another month in rather good health, driving his car, eating, etc. and then died. The pathologist performed autopsy and they found no malignancy.

The ears have a connection to the heart and "faith cometh by hearing and hearing by the word of God." While on the way to Damascus, God blinded Saul by a brilliant light SO THAT he could then hear from God. What we see with our physical eyes is only as real as we can actually see. What we do not see with our eyes, but with our hearts, is what really matters.

Doctors would be wise to inform patients that only God knows how long someone will live and we cannot prognosticate. They should say *"We've done all we know to do, but there are many people alive today who were told they were terminal. Don't give up! Don't lose hope!"* I have patients who were 'supposed to be' dead 5-10 years ago. They were terminally ill, yet are doing quite well.

Faith, Hope, and Charity (love of God) and the greatest is Charity. Science must find God before they can replace God by their faulty theories. First, you must love God, but in order to love God you must love yourself! When you love yourself, you will not defy God's dwelling place…your body! How do you love someone? You must learn to trust them by developing a relationship, by knowing the person.

The knowledge of God is what brings the power to have faith and heal. It is not only "belief" because our beliefs are not always right. Completely trusting in the object of your belief gives hope. Hope is what builds the faith. Science base our perceptions on our beliefs. When I have a very ill client, I tell them they must find the unseen benefit in their condition or healing can be very difficult. I tell them to write down as many benefits of having the condition, and then the negatives of the condition. If they cannot see the positive then they will probably never heal. I also tell them to write their obituary and epitaph. I tell them to write down goals for 1mo, 3mo, 6mo, 1yr and 2yrs and sign and date it with a witness. You must move past the fear of dying to heal, and people who do not do this usually do not heal. Obedience and the willingness to do anything to heal is the primary driving factor of faith. You are not trying, attempting, but choosing and determined to receive your miracle. You do not let family, friends, neighbors, doctors or anything keep you from your goal. Faith is holding on to nothing until it becomes something. It is the evidence of things not seen.

If you believe that the doctor is the final word, then you trust his or her diagnosis and study the disease to learn about it, but this reinforces all the symptoms connected to that valueless label. This brings in the fear of the unknown because you only have partial knowledge, not full knowledge.

When people see me, I do not tell them to do anything. I give them options. I am not responsible for their health. They are! I give them knowledge from my perspective and I tell them to inform themselves from the conventional side of medicine, as well as the natural side, and then decide which route to take. They should not rely on the people in their lives (spouse, friends, neighbor, dogcatcher, postal worker) to make the decision for them. They need to set boundaries by standing up for themselves and they will be empowered and more likely to heal.

People are constantly trying to solve other people's problems instead of their own because they feel neglected, rejected, and lack value in themselves. The primary character trait seen in people diagnosed with the label of "so called" Cancer is "People Pleaser and Peace Maker." They like to please other people, while the only people not pleased are themselves. At the heart level, they feel used! People have wounded them so many times that they have built walls around their heart to protect them.

I use the wrecking ball procedure to break down these walls. The person erects these walls prior to conception all the way to the present time. The younger you are, the more powerful the feelings are, and the more crucial is the need, for breaking down the walls. People will manipulate these "poor souls" and the only person that loses is the "poor soul." They build these walls on years of distrust, and the lack of nurturing and feeling loved. God helps you bring walls down so you can receive your healing.

How to make lasting change? First, you must set your intention (Goals). Write them down on a piece of paper and review them often.

Why do goals fail?

1. The person does not write the goals down, which means they have no power. A last will and testament means nothing if one does not write it down and have it witnessed. You need to write goals down and have a witness for accountability. It is amazing what this does to the heart in finding a solution to obtain these goals.

2. They are too lofty and unrealistic. If you were driving cross-country, would it be better to break it down into different segments of travel to make it easier? Surely, you might want to sleep at least one night.
3. No motivation.
4. No vehicle to get there (the process).
5. Goals set according to wants, not needs. Want equates to lack and the future, which never comes. The bible states in Philippians: *"My God will supply all your **needs** according to his riches and glory by Christ Jesus."* He did not say your wants.

Seven steps to Abundant Health

1. Have a purpose or meaning that is greater than yourself. We all have potential but potential is of no value until we put it into action. We all have possibilities and probability but these are of no value with discovering our value. We have to find the why and the how will take care of itself. We have to find the passion behind the purpose in our lives, which will promote the power needed to achieve anything.
2. Construct Social Boundaries with yourself, family, friends and others. When you do this, you will attract the right people for your journey through life and lose the manipulators. "So called" Cancer is mainly a lack of boundaries. Instead of doing the right thing and setting healthy boundaries, compromise wins the day. It is always about compromise.
3. Think first and then learn.
4. Education
5. Health
6. Work
7. Finances

You must have at least four of these things going for you or you will be unbalanced in your life and health.

Imagine your body is a tiny nation. The population is 100 trillion (cells) and you must budget to upkeep these poor souls. You must budget for feeding them quality food to eat. You must budget for the sanitation department to eliminate garbage and sewage. You must budget for chlorine and fluorine free water to their houses. You must budget for electricity to each house. You must budget for health care and dental care for each person. You must budget for the building and upkeep of the roads and bridges. You must budget to prevent terrorists from coming into your nation. We each have limited resources to keep our 100 trillion citizens happy and healthy. Make sure you are balancing the budget.

The sad fact is that most Americans do not take responsibility or accountability for their health. This is why only about 2% of us are enlightened to true health and the mainstream does not deceive us. Most people are looking for a free ride, but they place tremendous value and take great care of their material goods and possessions, while their health, which is most valuable, goes down the drain. The reason they do this is because the body cost them nothing, so that is the value they place on it.

This is not much different from the government. The government generates no money, but knows very well how to spend other people's money, and this is why America is almost 20 trillion dollars in debt. We must get our priorities right before humanity becomes extinct. It is all about "I"...I phone, I pad, I pod, Selfies. Selfishness is greed, not taking care of or loving each other.

First, we need to Love God. Then, we need to love ourselves and then, and only then, can we love others. People try to love others before they love themselves and then they only hate themselves. I have seen so many people absorb other people's problems and actually develop that person's physical issues themselves because of this lack of boundaries. You have to learn to do what is right, not the popular things in life. The road to what is right is usually the road that is less travelled and has many more weeds, rocks, and bumps along the way, but the benefits in the end are the greatest.

When the members at our lifestyle clinic evaluate issues in their lives, we discuss with them the concept of **RESTORATION: My Eleven Steps to Healing**

1. **Repent:** To have optimal healing of any condition, one first needs to be able to forgive self unconditionally, and then you will be able to forgive others. You must humble yourself and release yourself from the need to control anyone else. If you do not love yourself unconditionally without any strings attached, you will become a sponge for other people's issues. If you continue to go in the direction you are going, you will continue to get the same results. To repent basically means to make an about face. Turn from the way you are going and surrender your agenda. Submit, surrender, and release all your anger, resentment, bitterness, guilt and shame. Be completely willing to drop everything that holds you in bondage to unleash the miracle healing within. You must have death (repent) to your old way of living before restoration can occur.

2. **Exercise:** Not only is physical exercise, but also spiritual exercise. You must have a relationship with your Creator. This will allow you to have a relationship with His creation. How do we develop a relationship with our Creator? We have to develop as much knowledge as possible about Him by reading his word, meditating on his word, and doing his word. We are responsible not to only be hearers of the word, but also doers. Exercise requires doing, not just observing. When we have significant knowledge of our Creator, we will be able to trust him to unleash the miracle within.

3. **Sunlight:** Sunlight is extremely beneficial. It helps with Vitamin D production. It is a natural anti-depressant, helps restore the circadian rhythm, which allows for rest that is more efficient. The sunlight is anti-bacterial, anti-viral, anti-fungal and it is very cleansing.

4. **Thanksgiving:** We live in a thankless generation. Generally, people are only looking out for themselves and it is a dog eat dog

world. Optimally to heal, we need to be thankful for what we have instead of nurturing a needy attitude and a poverty mentality. We have our hands so full that nothing else will fit. We allow the media to tell us what we lack and they use the fear to manipulate us to buy things that we do not need. We are not producers anymore. We are the consumers. Society penalizes us for critical thinking and entrust people, businesses, and organizations we should not. God has given each of us talents and we should optimize, and be good stewards of those talents that God has granted us, instead of wishing we had other talents or possessions.

5. **Oxygen (Air):** Just go outside and breathe fresh air instead of toxic air inside our homes, vehicles, office etc. Last time I checked, air was still free.

6. **Rest:** People need at least 8 hours of sleep. There is a saying that every hour asleep prior to midnight is equivalent to 2 hours as far as healing is concerned. God places great value on Rest, so much so that even after the work that God did creating the universe, He rested. The first several hours of sleep are when we are in our deepest sleep, the cortisol levels are the lowest and the calming parasympathetic digesting hormones are the greatest. People who are trying to solve conflicts in their lives awaken around 3am and have difficulty returning to sleep. You should sleep in an environment that is comfortable, free of televisions, alarm clocks, EMF's, toxic chemicals, and geopathic disturbances. You should also take at least one day off per week to rest from your labor. When you get away from work, it allows you to recharge your batteries and improves your creativity.

7. **Adoration:** Praise God for what you possess AND what you do not possess. When you praise God, you promote the atmosphere where God can really work miracles in your life. If you leave the P off of Praise, then 'raise' is what you get. You must decrease in your life to be able to increase. You must give your life to gain your life. You must learn to die to some things in order to live. My father recently died and I was able to observe the dying process from start to finish. We monitored him with all types of equip-

ment at home and the thought came to me that really being a success in life is actually opposite of what society tells us. You must first learn to lose all your titles in life: (business owner or profession, property owner, employee, son or daughter, husband or wife, etc.) until one title remain, human being. When you relinquish all your titles, you will have no need to control. You must learn to trust others to the point that your dignity no longer matters. When you lose consciousness, you have no control over anything, so you have to learn to trust and not control. People literally hold on to things and never know the freedom of not controlling the outcome. In order to receive the healing that we need, begin by simply being a human being. Praise God because without Him, we have no being.

8. **Trust in God:** The hallmark

9. **Ins:** When we discuss ins, we are talking about the spiritual as well as physical. We must be discretionary about what we put into our bodies, as well as what we allow into our hearts. We have to take care of the temple of God, our bodies. We are spiritual beings living in physical bodies on this earth. If the body breaks down past the point of no return, then you must exit. We must take in the necessary amount of water (not including poisons such as sodas, coffee, highly caffeinated teas etc.)

    We must take great care to watch out for what we allow to come into our eyes and ears.

10. **Outs:** When we discuss outs, we are also talking about the spiritual as well as physical. You must have necessary output and monitor your urine and bowel movements. You should have at least two bowel movements per day that are not difficult to pass. Your urine should be clear, light in color, and free of smell (unless of course you have eaten some asparagus!)

    You must observe the words you say to yourself and others. The bible says, *"It is not what goes in that defiles a man but what comes out of his mouth."* With God's help, we need to be careful to tame our tongues.

11. **Nutrition:** The only part of my plan that has a financial cost. It is

really more of an investment, because it could save you a tremendous amount of money in the long term. You have to look always at the long-term investment instead of short term. It really pays off to be healthy.

I conclude this book with two of my favorite Voltaire quotes:

1. "The art of medicine consists of amusing the patient while nature cures the disease."
2. "Doctors are men who prescribe medicines of which they know little, to cure disease of which they know less, in human beings of whom they know nothing."

I am a medical entertainer, who knows very little, but I know the God of the Universe and He knows everything.

*   *   *

For more information, email me at tlucky_1@yahoo.com

Made in the
USA
Monee, IL